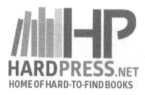

Consumption: Its Prevention and Cure by the Water Treatment
by Joel Shew

T B Carpen
157 Orange
New

FOWLERS AND WELLS'

WATER-CURE LIBRARY,

Embracing

ALL THE MOST POPULAR WORKS

ON THE SUBJECT:

INCLUDING:

INTRODUCTION TO THE WATER-CURE;
HYDROPATHY, OR THE WATER-CURE;
EXPERIENCE IN THE WATER-CURE;
THE CHOLERA, AND BOWEL DISEASES;
WATER AND VEGETABLE DIET;
THE PARENTS' GUIDE;
TOBACCO: ITS NATURE AND EFFECTS;

CURIOSITIES OF COMMON WATER;
WATER-CURE MANUAL;
WATER-CURE IN EVERY DISEASE;
WATER-CURE IN PREGNANCY;
HYDROPATHY FOR THE PEOPLE;
ERRORS IN THE WATER-CURE;
WATER-CURE IN CONSUMPTION.

IN SEVEN VOLUMES.

VOL. VII.

WATER-CURE IN CONSUMPTION;
WATER-CURE IN PREGNANCY.

NEW YORK:

FOWLERS AND WELLS, PUBLISHERS,
NO. 308 BROADWAY.

SOLD BY BOOKSELLERS GENERALLY

CONSUMPTION:

ITS PREVENTION AND CURE

BY THE

WATER TREATMENT.

WITH ADVICE CONCERNING

HÆMORRHAGE·FROM THE LUNGS, COUGHS, COLDS,
ASTHMA, BRONCHITIS, AND SORE THROAT.

BY JOEL SHEW, M. D.
PRACTITIONER OF WATER-CURE.

NEW YORK:
FOWLERS AND WELLS, PUBLISHERS,
NO. 308 BROADWAY.

BOSTON:
142 Washington St.

1855.

PHILADELPHIA:
No. 231 Arch Street.

INTRODUCTION.

In addition to what has been said concerning diet, as a means of prevention and cure of consumption, and its kindred diseases, in the work now presented to the public, the author wishes here to call more especial attention to the subject.

The common belief among the civilized and enlightened nations of the earth, is, that man is, by nature, an *omnivorous*, or all-eating animal; that, in a state of pure nature, if such a state can be conceived of, he eats naturally, and with benefit, of flesh, fish, fowl, farinacea, fruits, and roots, according to his inclination, and the circumstances in which he is placed. The practice of the civilized world is in accordance with its belief, with this exception, that in many parts, as, for example, France and Germany, the poorer portion of the population, which also constitutes by far the most numerous part, must of necessity subsist almost entirely on the vegetable productions of the earth. It may, indeed, be stated, that the manual labor of the world is done mainly on the strength gained from vegetable food. But this practice arises merely from the necessity of the case. The poor are not able to obtain animal food, because of its scarcity, and higher price.

If we look at man in the light of comparative anatomy, we find that his teeth do not at all resemble those of the omnivorous hog, or of any other omnivorous animal we can find. True, he has what is called a canine tooth; but this is merely a transition from the double to the single teeth, and is possessed by other animals, which are well known to be herbivorous, equally with man. On the other hand, too,

we find that the orang-outang, the animal which, in all respects of anatomical conformation, nearest resembles man,
has the same number and order of teeth, and the jaw and
teeth of which may be readily mistaken for those of the human species.   If we extend our observation to other organs
of the body, we also find a striking resemblance between
the orang-outang and man.   The orang-outang, it is well
known, is never, in a natural state, in any sense omnivorous.
He eats only of the vegetable productions of the earth.

The great objections to animal food, in a physiological
point of view, are these : it causes too rapid circulation, and
too great heat of the system ; it increases its tendency to
inflammatory action, and thus renders it, at all times, more
liable to the attacks of disease ; it over-stimulates the powers of life, and tends preternaturally to wear out the energies of the living body, and thus to shorten man's days.

It is common, I know, with many to recommend to feeble
patients more stimulating and highly concentrated food.
But this is done on the blind supposition that the enfeebled stomach is able to digest such food.   As well might
we give a feeble horse a greater burden, and expect him to
bear it, as to attempt to goad on the energies of the system, by giving it a greater than ordinary task to perform.
The feebler the system, always the less able is it to digest
food.   In other words, the amount of food must always be
graduated in proportion to the strength of the individual.

The *quantity* of food, then, is a most important matter.
In the treatment of the more active and later stages of consumption, we often see people partaking freely of the richest viands, under the supposition that the stomach is well
enough off.   So great is the disease going on in the lungs,
the stomach cannot at all *feel* the mischiefs it is brought to
endure.   The law of the system is, that when a strong disease is at work in any one organ of the body, the other parts
remain in a comparatively dormant state.   But in all such
cases, the weak and diseased organ receives the injury of
the offending cause.   Thus, in the case supposed, the abuses
of the stomach are sent upon the lungs.

Patients in an advanced state of pulmonary disease, will
always find that if, in connection with other well-regulated

and judicious means, they practice a good degree of abstinence in food, their bad symptoms will uniformly become
mitigated ; they will find that they have less feverishness,
less debility and sweats, less diarrhœa, less cough and expectoration, and that they will enjoy better sleep at night.
If free, regular, and continued exercise, in the open air, is
to be regarded the great remedy of preventing consumption, in its earliest stages, I am convinced that abstinence,
carried almost to the point of living on simple water, is the
greatest of all known means for mitigating its symptoms,
in its latter and more painful periods.

I have known a case like the following : a woman about
thirty years of age, with many of the most formidable symptoms of deep-seated pulmonary consumption, such as severe
cough, the raising of large quantities of very offensive expectoration, wasting of the flesh, total loss of appetite, hectic, night sweats, extreme debility, cessation of the menses,
etc., to become cured in this simple way : she was kept for
months nearly fasting ; ocasionally as the appetite returned
somewhat, a little mild nourishment was given her, but the
appetite was never urged ; at length she grew slightly better, and thus by going on little by little, as appetite returned, living yet all the time in a most abstemious manner,
she, after many months, became well. Now in this case
it must be considered, I think, that the prolonged fasting
and abstemiousness broke up her disease. And it was accomplished in this wise ; under wasting, caused by lack of
food, the tendency of the system is to throw off its morbid,
diseased, and worn-out matter first. This is, indeed, the
tendency of nature always, but to a much greater degree
when prolonged fasting from all food is practiced. I have
no doubt that consumption in numbers of cases, and other
so-called incurable diseases, might in this way be eradicated. The *hunger-cure*, as it is called in Germany, acts on
the principle just explained. "I am convinced by every
day's experience," says Laennec, "that for one instance of
mischief produced by too great abstinence in the convalescence from acute, and especially from inflammatory diseases, there are a thousand occasioned by the opposite
extreme. And I would, therefore," he continues, "earnestly

request the young practitioner not to be seduced into the too early exhibition of nutritive food to his convalescents, from fear of dangerous debility, or any other cause."

On the other hand, it should be remembered, too, that there is such a thing as carrying fasting too far. A sick man may be starved as easily and as effectually as one that is well. The error is, however, almost always on the side of too great an amount of food.

The subject of diet, being a most important one, not only as regards the prevention and cure of consumption, but of all diseases whatever, I earnestly recommend the reader to avail himself of such works as Dr. Lambe on Vegetable Diet, Dr. Alcott, and Mr. Graham's Science of Human Life. These works contain a vast deal of general and practical information, and such as will amply reward the reader, even if he do not become convinced of all the positions laid down by these authors.

In cases of *colds in the chest and lungs, bronchitis, cough, and common sore throat*, the treatment recommended by Priessnitz is both simple and efficacious. Mr. Henry C. Wright, whose case as cured at Graefenberg, is given in this volume, obtained of Priessnitz his advice to be followed, in the attacks to which he had for years been liable. The questions and answers, as Mr. Wright gives them in his "Six Months at Graefenberg," are as follows:

" *Wright.*—In case of severe cold on the lungs, attended with much cough and expectoration, what should be done?

" *Priessnitz.*—Rub the chest and throat with cold water, holding, at the same time, some water in the mouth. In cold climates, the wet bandage around the throat would be of service occasionally. In warm climates, washing and rubbing alone are better.

" *Wright.*—In cases of inflammation and soreness of the throat, attended with hoarseness and difficulty in speaking?

" *Priessnitz.*—Friction, washing, and the application of wet bandages.

" *Wright.*—In cases of long attendance, and speaking at public meetings, in hot, close, crowded rooms, and then going out into the chilly night air?

"*Priessnitz.*—The rubbing-sheet, washing and rubbing the head and throat well, and the use of the foot-bath.

"*Wright.*—When troubled with shooting pains across the chest, occasioned by long speaking at a time?

"*Priessnitz.*—Take rubbing-sheets, and rub the throat and chest with water.'

In regard to friction, Mr. Wright judiciously remarks, "that it is worthy of special notice that Priessnitz never orders the rubbing to be done with brushes, flannels, or linen towels. He never applies flannels and brushes to the skin for any purpose; linen is only used for wiping the surface dry, and, even in this process, the rubbing should be gentle. He wishes to have the skin kept as smooth and soft as possible; and hence his disuse of flannels next the skin, and of brushes and hard substances in rubbing. He recommends that the hand only should be used; and it is not possible to be long under his treatment, and to enjoy the delicious sensations resulting from a clear, smooth, soft skin, the almost invariable result of the cure, without being convinced of the correctness of his practice in this respect."

The free use of the dripping-sheet (rubbing *over* the sheet, and not *with* it, for four or five minutes, until it becomes warm) is a most valuable remedy in colds and recent affections of the throat and chest. It is the most mild of all general baths, and can be obtained in almost any circumstances in which we may be placed.

In cases of old and chronic affections of the throat, the water-treatment, together with suitable diet and exercise, long persevered in, will be found a most serviceable means, and, in fact, the only means that will in the end accomplish any thing in their cure. The fashionable practice of clipping the tonsils and palate, and applying a solution of nitrate of silver to the throat, will be found of very little benefit. In some cases, it may relieve the symptoms somewhat for the time; but in the end, all such treatment must prove worse than nothing. It does not at all go to the root of the difficulty. The only cure of a chronic throat affection is the complete renovation of the whole system. The throat too, be it remembered, as an important practical lesson, is, in such cases the very last part to become benefited.

Clergymen, and all others, who are troubled with this most obstinate affection, are earnestly recommended to make themselves acquainted with the water-treatment.

In *asthma*, this same treatment will be found of most signal benefit. It was long ago observed, by Mr. Wesley and other writers, that the cold bath was a very efficacious remedy in this obstinate disease. A single cold bath will often relieve a person as by magic, when he is nearly suffocating from want of breath.

In *hooping-cough*, the water processes are of great service. No treatment can at all compare with that by wet compresses on the chest, the dripping-sheet, frictions with the wet hand, cold general baths, if the patient is not too weak, water drinking, and reasonable abstinence in food. Indeed, the same treatment we use for a common cold, will be strictly applicable in this affection.

The author has not, in the following pages, spoken of *percussion* and *auscultation*, as means of ascertaining the state of the chest and lungs, in consumption. These are complex and difficult methods, and are moreover liable to mislead. They may serve to amuse the patient, and bring money to the physician; but as to their real worth, there is but little in them. We know that the most experienced often vary in their opinions of a given case; and if it were possible (which it is not) to learn by these means, in all cases, the true state of the parts concerned, it would not help us one iota in the treatment. The true and rational treatment of consumption must always be that which is graduated according to the patient's strength. Percussion and auscultation do not, in the least, aid us in ascertaining what the degree of strength is. It does not help us in any mode of treatment whatever.

CONTENTS.

CHAPTER XIV.

CHAPTER XV.

CHAPTER XVI.

CHAPTER XVII.

CHAPTER XVIII.

CHAPTER XIX.

CHAPTER XX.

CHAPTER XXI.

CHAPTER XXII.

CHAPTER XXIII.

CONSUMPTION.

CHAPTER I.

Consumption.—Meaning of the word.—Its derivation and application.—Signification of Phthisis Pulmonalis.—Dr. Hooper's seven varieties of consumption.—True meaning of the term at the present day.—Consumption a disease that belongs to all ages, and all classes of individuals.—It extends over a wide range of the earth's surface. —It is more to be feared than any other disease which afflicts the race.—Consumption is often, though not always, an hereditary disease.—Persons of a particular conformation and habit of body more liable than others to the disease.

THE word CONSUMPTION—from *consumere*, to waste away—in its most extended signification, as applied to the living body, denotes that progressive emaciation which usually precedes death in the most of chronic diseases. The appellation is, however, more commonly used to designate a *scrofulous ulceration* of the lungs. By consumption, as used in this country at the present day, is generally understood a *wasting away of the substance of the lungs*. *Phthisis*, from a Greek word signifying to consume, and *pulmonalis* (from pulmo, the lung) is the medical term for the same affection. *Phthisis* alone is often used ; *pulmonalis* being understood.

Dr. Hooper, in his medical dictionary, makes seven varieties of consumption :

CONSUMPTION.

1. *Phthisis incipiens,* incipient consumption, without an expectoration of pus.

2. *Phthisis humida,* consumption with an expectoration of pus.

3. *Phthisis scrophulosa,* consumption from scrofulous tubercles of the lungs.

4. *Phthisis hæmoptoica,* consumption from hæmoptysis, or hæmorrhage from the lungs.

5. *Phthisis exanthematica,* consumption from exanthemata, or eruptive diseases.

6. *Phthisis chlorotica,* consumption from chlorosis of females.

7. *Phthisis syphilitica,* consumption from venereal ulceration of the lungs.

Phthisis signifies, as I have said, *a wasting away,* or *a consuming* of the body ; but of late years the term has been restricted to that species of wasting which is caused by the presence of tubercular matter in the lungs. But it would be an error to suppose that the disease is restricted to the lungs in this case. The lung disease would indeed, of itself, be sufficient, in most cases, to destroy life ; but its mortal tendency is aided and accelerated, in most instances, by diseases of a similar character situated in other organs. " The *pulmonary* consumption," as Dr. Latham justly observes, "is no more than a fragment of a great constitutional malady ;" but that malady plays its part most conspicuously in the lungs.

Consumption is a disease belonging to all classes of individuals. No age is exempt from its ravages. The unborn child has been found affected with it, and it is extremely common among the children of the poorer classes in large cities, as is proved by the records of hospitals and other charitable institutions for the young. It invades the system also at the age when childhood is passing into adolescence, and not less frequently when the system is at the period of its greatest maturity and strength. From the fortieth to the fiftieth year it is frequent, and old age is by no means exempt from it. Even at the advanced period of one hundred years, persons have died of tuberculous pulmonary disease.

"Consumption," in the language of an able writer —Professor Sweetser—"may be traced back to the earliest periods of medical history. Hippocrates, commonly styled the father of medicine, who lived more than four hundred years before the Christian era, knew it, and has well described its melancholic course ; and though ages have rolled on with all their changes, this bane of human life still remains the same—has never abated in its fatality—never rested in its work of destruction. No condition, no period of human life, can claim immunity from its ravages. It respects not station, for it is a disease equally of the rich and the poor. It attacks childhood in its weakness, youth in its bloom and elasticity, manhood in its power, and age in its decrepitude."

Consumption is a disease which extends itself over a wide range of the earth's surface. In all northern Europe, in the United States, and in temperate climates generally, this disease is more to be feared than any other which afflicts our race.

In many instances we find that consumption is evidently an hereditary affection. The universal experience of physicians proves that children of consumptive parents are more subject to it than others are. It is true that we fortunately find exceptions to this rule; but these exceptions are enough only to prove the general fact. "We sometimes find families," observes Laennec, "in which only one or two of their members become consumptive in each generation; on the other hand, we sometimes find large families of children destroyed by consumption, whose parents had showed no signs of the disease."

Persons of a particular temperament or constitution are the most subject to consumption. This particular habit of the body, is distinguished by "the brilliant whiteness of the skin, the bright red of the cheeks, the narrowness of the chest, the projecting or winged configuration of the shoulder-blades, and the slenderness of the limbs and trunk, which is, at the same time, combined with a certain degree of adipose and lymphatic stoutness." Aretæus, however, attributed this particular constitution rather to hæmoptysical than consumptive subjects; but it is to be remarked, as Laennec observes, "that consumptive subjects of this configuration, are more subject to hæmoptysis (hæmorrhage from the lungs) than others." It is to be observed also, that individuals of this particular constitution form only the smaller proportion of consumptive patients, and that this terrible malady frequently cuts off those who are the most robust, and have the best bodily configuration.

CHAPTER II.

Females are, more than males, subject to consumption.—This is evidently not the natural order of things.—Reasons why males are less subject to pulmonary disease.—Opinion of Dr. Forbes.—Dr. Sweetser.—The Parisian hospitals.—Tables of mortality.—Scrofula also more common among females.—How are we to account for the fact that females are more subject to scrofulous disease?

WHEN we examine the facts on an extended scale, it appears evident that women are decidedly more subject to consumption than males. It cannot, I think be supposed that the Creator, in infinite wisdom, and in the beautiful fitness of things every where to be observed in nature, would have ordered such a result. It is said, I know, that woman has naturally a greater delicateness of constitution, and that she is less able to bear up against the physical ills of life. But are we not rather to attribute this fact to the faulty methods of female life; as Dr. Forbes remarks, " to their most deleterious system of physical education, from the age of ten to puberty—to the wearing of stays, and the exposure of the upper part of the chest ?" May we not also take into this account the fact that in all nations, and in all periods of time, a very nearly equal number of each sex have been found to exist ? We cannot, I infer, suppose that the one sex was originally created with any greater *natural* predisposition to this disease than the other.

From the tables I have quoted in another part of this work—those of M. Benoiston de Chateauneuf—it appears that in Paris males are less subject to consumption than females. "The reports of the Paris hospitals," says Dr. Sweetser, "which are on a very extended scale, and made by the most scientific and accurate medical observers of France, unite in proving a greater relative mortality from consumption in females than among males." Louis, whose observations were perhaps as much extended as those of any one, states the proportion as seventy to ninety-two. Dr. Clark, of England, also exhibits tables, drawn from the medico-statistical reports of different countries, but which show a result somewhat different from the statement of Louis, but yet in favor of males. M. Benoiston's tables, it will be seen by referring to them, give, as the results of four of the Parisian hospitals—the L'Hotel-Dieu, La Charite, La Pitie, and L'Hospice Cochin—during ten years, 4.77 per centum of deaths of females, while of males there died but 2.85 per centum.

M. Louis, as quoted by Sir James Clark, found in his practice, that among females there were, during the first year, *forty-two* deaths to *thirty* of males. After this, the ratio of mortality as to time was the same in both sexes.

Dr. Clark has given a table, gleaned from the records of different cities, showing a result somewhat different from the conclusions of some other writers. The table, taken in the aggregate, however, shows females to be the more subject to the disease. It is as follows :

	Males.	Females.	Proportions.
Hamburgh	555	445	10 to 8.7
Rouen Hospital (in France)	55	44	10 to 8.6
Naples Hospital	382	315	10 to 8.2
New York	1584	1370	10 to 8.6
Geneva	71	62	10 to 8.7
Berlin	328	292	10 to 8.8
Sweden	2088	1860	10 to 8.9
Ditto.	3054	3103	10 to 10.4
Berlin	560	655	10 to 11.6
Blacks, New York	47	58	10 to 12.3
Paris	2219	2970	10 to 13.3
Ditto.	3965	5579	10 to 14.3
Berlin, boys and girls	363	567	10 to 15.6

Scrofula, which is also a kindred disease of consumption, appears to affect females more than males, in different parts of the world. Thus that peculiar swelling of the throat called bronchocele (*goitre* is the common name), which is supposed to be a scrofulous disease, is found to be more common with women than men. "It prevails," says Dr. Sweetser, "in some districts of our own country, as on certain parts of the Connecticut river, and on the borders of some of our northern lakes; but is seen on a vastly more extended scale among the Alps, and other mountainous ranges of Europe, as the Apennines and Pyrenees. In some situations among the Alps, goitre is so common as to seem almost a local characteristic. But wherever I have had opportunities of observing the affection, I have remarked females to be its more frequent subjects." The same thing is seen, only probably to a less extent, along the Sudates of Silesia, Austria, among which mountains the far-famed Water-Cure establishment of Priessnitz is situated.

If, then, it is true that females are more subject to consumption, and its kindred diseases, than males—a fact which cannot be doubted—how are we to assign a reason for this apparent anomaly in nature? Are we to believe that the Almighty Disposer of all human events would thus create one half of the race with constitutions more subject to a malady so fearful as this? Who can believe it? I, for one, would much rather look carefully, reverently, into the ways of man's physical wrong-doing for a solution of this question—a question in which every member of society is interested.

Is it said of females, as I have already hinted, that their native softness and delicacy of structure approximate them more nearly to that physical condition which tends strongly to scrofula and tubercular disease? that this dainty organization of the female economy seems incompatible with that free energy of life which is needful to react against those vicissitudes of climate so operative in the generation of tubercles?

Are we not rather to say, that the habits of females generally, throughout the civilized world, are, and for centuries have been, such as are calculated, in no small degree, to waste, through successive generations, the inherent energies of the female frame? Thus the disease is augmented in both sexes, but most in those who transgress the laws of nature to the greatest extent.

CHAPTER III.

Periods of life at which consumption is most apt to occur.—Doctrine of the Greeks.—Table of M. Louis; of Laennec; of Dr. Alison; of Sussmilah; of M. Bayle, as quoted by M. Louis; of Dr. Clark.

It was a common doctrine among the Greek physicians that consumption rarely occurs before fifteen or after thirty-five years of age; and the opinion of most practitioners at the present day seems to be very much in accordance with this. I have remarked elsewhere that it may occur at any age, and even in the unborn child. Yet certain periods of life are more subject to it. Between the ages of eighteen and thirty-five the larger proportion of deaths occur but there are in this country at the present time a much larger proportion of deaths occurring after thirty or thirty-five years of age from consumption than is generally supposed.

A table of M. Louis showing the ages at which death occurs from consumption is as follows:

From 15 to 20 years of age,............... 11 deaths.
" 20 " 30 " " .... 39 "
" 30 " 40 ' " .... 33 "
" 40 " 50 ' " .... 23 "
" 50 " 60 " " .... 12 "
" 60 " 70 " " .... 5 "

In a table of Laennec of 223 deaths from consumption, recorded by Bayle and Louis, there were—

From 15 to 20 years of age,............. 21 deaths.
 "   20 " 30   "   "   62   "
 "   30 " 40   "   "   56   "
 "   40 " 50   "   "   44   "
 "   50 " 60   "   "   27   "
 "   60 " 70   "   "   13   "

Dr. Alison gives, as the result of practice in the New Town Dispensary, at Edinburgh, 55 deaths occurring during the two years, as follows:

Before 15 years of age, ... 8 deaths.
From 15 to 30 years of age,............. 13   "
 "   30 " 40   "   "   10   "
After 40   "   "   24   "

A table of Sussmilah, of Berlin, made in 1746, is as follows:

Before 15 years of age,................. 251 deaths.
From 15 to 30 years of age,............. 73   "
 "   30 " 40   "   "   66   "
Above 40   "   "   230   "

Louis has given, also, another table, on the authority of M. Bayle, as follows:

From 15 to 20 years of age,............. 10 deaths.
 "   20 " 30   "   "   23   "
 "   30 " 40   "   "   33   "
 "   40 " 50   "   "   21   "
 "   50 " 60   "   "   15   "
 "   60 " 70   "   "   8   "

Dr. Clark has collected two tables, from observations made in different cities and countries, the general average of which goes to show that the greatest number of deaths from consumption occurs between the ages of twenty and thirty. Next in proportion, between thirty and forty, and next between forty and fifty. This remarkable agreement of all the places of observation warrants the conclusion, that after the fifteenth year of age fully one half of the deaths from consumption occur between the twentieth and fortieth, and that mortality is about at its maximum at thirty—and from that time gradually diminishes.

CHAPTER IV.

Duration of consumption, and seasons of the year in which it is most prevalent.—It is generally a slow or chronic disease.—Testimony of M. Bayle and M. Louis.—Their tables, showing the duration of the disease.—This depends on a variety of circumstances.—Observations of M. Louis and Dr. Clark.—Season of the year as affecting the duration of consumption.—Dr. Heberden's Bills of Mortality in the city of London, as quoted by Dr. Clark on this point.—City Inspector's Report of Deaths and Interments in the city of New York.—Comparative mortality of males and females at different seasons of the year.

CONSUMPTION, like all other diseases, varies much in regard to its progress. It is essentially a chronic disease; although in some cases persons die in a very short period after its invasion, and in which it takes on more the form of an acute disease.

According to the tables of Bayle and Louis, from observations concerning 314 fatal cases, the average duration of the disease was twenty-three months. Counting from the time when consumption becomes fairly seated upon the system, the mean duration of cases may be stated at two years. This was Andral's conclusion. Many, of course, die in a much shorter period.

The following are the tables of Louis and Bayle, referred to above:

					Louis. 8 cases.		Bayle. 16 cases.		Total, 24	
Deaths	within	3	months,	"	25	"	44	"	"	69
" from	3	to	6	"	25	"	44	"	"	69
" from	6	to	9	"	25	"	44	"	"	69
" from	9	to	12	"	12	"	20	"	"	32
" from	12	to	15	"	12	"	21	"	"	33
" from	15	to	18	"	3	"	9	"	"	12
" from	18	to	24	"	10	"	18	"	"	28
" from	3	to	5 years,	14	"	14	"	"		28
" from	5	to	10	"	1	"	9	"	"	10
" from	10	to	40	"	4	"	5	"	"	9
					114		200			314

It should be borne in mind that these tables are calculated from fatal cases, which occurred in hospital practice.

The duration of consumption depends upon a variety of circumstances. The constitution, the general health of the individual, the age, sex, occupation, season of the year, climate, and external circumstances, all have their influence. According to Louis—who is certainly very high authority on this subject—very acute cases are more frequent in early life ; but Dr. Clark tells us that his own experience in this respect differs from that of Louis, for whose opinion he has great regard.

" In the upper ranks of society," says Dr. Clark, "where patients have all the advantages that the best regimen, change of air, and medical treatment can afford, the medium duration of consumption is probably not much short of three years. Under other circumstances it is less." "And it is melancholical to reflect," says this estimable authority, " that cures occur in so small a ratio, that in estimating the duration of this disease we cannot bring them into the calculation."

Season of the year as affecting the duration of consumption.—That the duration of consumption is greatly influenced by the seasons, appears by the following table, compiled by Dr. Clark, from the particulars given in Dr. Heberden's Bills of Mortality, which show the distribution of deaths from this disease, through the different months of the year, in the city of London.

In January,	4,363	deaths.
In February,	4,527	"
In March,	4,634	"
In April,	4,227	"
In May,	4,043	"
In June,	3,604	"
In July,	3,242	"
In August,	2,825	"
In September,	2,994	"
In October,	3,521	"
In November,	3,711	"
In December,	4,516	"

The result of this table accords with the common observation, that the disease proves more fatal in the cold months than in the warm According to the seasons, the aggregate number will stand thus :

Winter months,	13,406	deaths.
Spring months,	12,904	"
Autumnal months,	10,226	"
Summer months,	9,678	"

According to the City Inspector's Annual Report of the number of deaths and interments in the city of New York, during the different months of the year

1848, we find the number of deaths occurring from consumption as stated below :

January,	215 deaths.
February,	202 "
March,	182 "
April,	150 "
May,	147 "
June,	126 "
July,	146 "
August,	147 "
September,	121 "
October,	156 "
November,	129 "
December,	148 "

This table, it will be seen, shows a corresponding result of observations between the cities of **London** and New York.

That the inclement seasons of the year are more productive of consumption than the mild would also appear from the fact that males, who are more than females exposed to the changes of temperature, storms, and the like influences, have a greater relative mortality in cold seasons. This will appear from the following particulars, gleaned from the City Inspector's Report of deaths and interments in the city of **New** York, for the year as above :

January,	116 males,	and	99 females.
February,	105 "		99 "
March,	91 "		91 "
April,	80 "		70 "
May,	80 "		67 "
June,	62 "		64 "
July,	65 "		81 "
August,	70 "		77 "

2*

September,.................... 59 males, and 62 females.
October,...................... 77   "   79   "
November,.................... 70   "   59   "
December,.................... 73   "   75   "*

It should not, however, be inferred from this table, that because consumption is more prevalent in the city of New York in the cold seasons, it would necessarily be advantageous to remove to a warmer climate. In the latter there are other influences than mere warmth to be taken into the account. We know that consumption is very rare, almost unknown in Northern Russia. We know, also, that in some warm climates it is very prevalent. But a temporary change from one place to another is doubtless often beneficial.

* This table, showing that more males than females die of consumption in the city of New York, might at first appear to exhibit a result different from that which I have elsewhere stated, namely, that females are more subject than males to this disease. But it should be remembered that because of the more transient character of a considerable portion of the population of this city, and because of the fact that more of males than females are engaged in city pursuits, we are to infer that there is always, necessarily, in this city, a greater number of the former than of the latter. Hence this result.

CHAPTER V.

Mortality of consumption.—Imperfect nature of statistical reports.—
These are, however, sufficient for all practical purposes.—Number
of deaths occurring, and at what ages, in the city of New York.—
Also, the number from each disease.—Conclusions drawn there-
from.—Estimate of Dr. Sydenham of deaths by consumption
in Great Britain.—Of Drs. Heberden, Young, and Woolcombe.—
Great amount of consumption in Bristol, England.—Laennec's estimate concerning Paris.—Dr. Sweetser's estimate of consumption
in the city of Boston.—Dr. Elliotson's statement concerning
Europe.—Dr. Emerson's estimate in the American cities.—Mortality among the English troops stationed in different parts of the
world.—Conclusions drawn from the foregoing facts.

In order that some definite idea may be gained respecting the fearfulness of the disease under consideration, I will present the reader with some items of
statistical information, which, however, it must be admitted are always to a greater or less degree inaccu-
rate, and not from any want of honesty in those who
make such reports, but from the great difficulties
which always necessarily belong to calculations of
the kind. Still, such calculations are sufficiently accurate to enable us to arrive at an approximation of
the truth.

According to the New York City Inspector's Annual Report of 1848, the deaths during the year previous were as follows:

Whole number of deaths,....................... 15,788
Of children under 5 years of age,............... 7,373
   "   "   between 5 and 10 years of age,..... 571
Of those between 10 and 20   "   " 646
 "   "   "   20 " 30   "   " 1,947
 "   "   "   30 " 40   "   " 1,833
 "   "   "   40 " 50   "   " 1,279
 "   "   "   50 " 60   "   " 746
 "   "   "   60 " 70   "   " 580
 "   "   "   70 " 80   "   " 389
 "   "   "   80 " 90   "   " 153
 "   "   "   90 " 100   "   " 35
                  Above 100   "   " 3

The principal diseases of the mortality of this year, and the number of deaths from each, are stated as below :

Typhus and typhoid fever,........................ 1,396
Apoplexy,....................................... 446
Cholera infantum,............................... 692
Convulsions,.................................... 1,023
Debility,....................................... 515
Dropsy of the head,............................. 559
Croup,.. 274
Erysipelas,..................................... 162
Measles,.. 275
Scarlet fever,.................................. 142
Old age,.. 180
Delirium tremens,............................... 137
Small pox,...................................... 53
Whooping cough,................................. 86
Cholera morbus,................................. 44
Inflammation of the lungs,...................... 748
Consumption,.................................... 1,926

Thus we see, according to this Report, that of the diseases of this metropolis, much the largest number

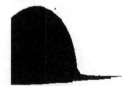

of deaths occurred from consumption. And if **we** deduct the number of deaths that occurred in persons under twenty years of age, before which death very seldom occurs from this disease, and at the same time bear in mind the fact that probably a considerable number of those reported as dying from "debility," actually died from pulmonary consumption, we are led to the conclusion, that of all adults dying in the city of New York, more than *one fourth* is from this dire disease. It must, however, be admitted that medical reports, as made at the present day, are, in the aggregate, always, to a greater or less extent, incorrect. But we may safely infer from those of the city of New York, that, year by year, when no great epidemic, like the cholera, prevails, *about one fourth of all deaths occurring after puberty are from pulmonary consumption.*

The ratio of deaths by consumption in the city of New York during this year (1848), in proportion to the *whole* number of deaths, is a little less than one in eight, a result somewhat different from what has been arrived at in the statistics of other cities of the Union, and of the same city in other years.

According to Dr. Sydenham, two thirds of those who died of chronic disease in Great Britain, fell victims to consumption. The estimates of Drs. Heberden, Young, and Woolcombe show us that an average of about one in four of the deaths which happen in Great Britain are from this disease.

It is said to be a curious fact, that in Bristol, England, there is the greatest relative amount of mortality from consumption, and among its native inhabitants, too, of any place yet compared with it; although this town is in the southern part of the country, and is a great and popular resort for consumptive patients from other parts. This fact does not, certainly, speak very well for the judgment of those who send them thither.

" Laennec states," says Dr. Sweetser, "that in Paris, and the great cities in the interior of France, the proportion of deaths from consumption is well known to be one in four or five."

In the city of Boston, according to Dr. Sweetser, " the average number of deaths by consumption, as compared with other diseases, may be about one in four or five. In New York, the proportion will vary but little from this. In Philadelphia, it may be about one in five."

Dr. Elliotson quotes Dr. Thomas Young (author of a Practical and Historical Treatise on Consumptive Diseases, whom the former regards as good authority, he having referred to every work written on the subject previously to his own), as asserting that one fourth of the inhabitants of Europe die of consumption.

Dr. Emerson, of Philadelphia, states the relative number of deaths by consumption in the larger cities of the United States as being, in proportion to the whole mortality, as follows :

In New York,... 1 in 5.23
" Boston,... 1 " 5.54
" Baltimore,.. 1 " 6.21
" Philadelphia,..................................... 1 " 6.38

The number of deaths, in proportion to the whole population, in the different cities, according to this author's estimate, are:

In New York,............................... 1 in 39.36
" Baltimore,................................ 1 " 39.17
" Boston,.................................. 1 " 44.93
" Philadelphia,............................. 1 " 47.86

A table, showing the proportion of deaths from all diseases, and also from consumption among English troops as stationed at different parts of the world, has been given by Dr. Clark, from which the following is an abstract. The basis of reckoning is one thousand men. The numbers show the proportion of deaths from all diseases, and how many from consumption per thousand in one year:

Where stationed.	All diseases.	Consumpt.
East Indies and New South Wales,..........	57.5	1.1
Cape of Good Hope,......................	14.5	1.6
Western Coast of Africa,...................	144.5	1.7
Mauritius,..............................	28.2	3.2
West Indies (Europeans),..................	80.3	4.9
West Indies (Negroes),...................	26.6	13.7
Bermudas,..............................	12.4	2.3
Canadas and Nova Scotia,.................	12.2	3.4
Malta...................................	14.7	2.6
Gibraltar,...............................	13.1	2.4
Ionian Islands...........................	26.6	2.1
Malta, Portugal, Gibraltar, and Ionian Islands,.	24.2	1.6
City of London, 1820 to 1830,.............	19	6.2

From this table it appears that the average of about one in ten of deaths of English troops is from consumption. It is however, to be remembered that military men are chosen from among the most healthy and hardy of the inhabitants, and that, too, from males, who are on the whole least subject to this disease.

We have no registry of deaths in this country, as in Great Britain, except in the larger cities. It is, therefore, impossible for us to tell whether consumption is more prevalent, according to the whole number of deaths, in the city or country. Probably, there is more of it in proportion to the number of inhabitants in the former than in the latter.

From the foregoing facts, it appears that in the most enlightened parts of the world, from one fourth to one eighth of all deaths are caused by that greatest bane of human life, tubercular consumption. It is a most insidious malady, coming upon us like a thief in the night, so stealthily, indeed, that in most instances, neither the patient nor his friends, and often not even his physician, are aware of the true nature of the case, until it is absolutely too late to attempt any thing more than mere palliation of the disease.

CHAPTER VI.

Anatomical description of the chest and lungs.—The thorax, or chest.
—The lungs.—Their situation, color, divisions, size, number of
lobes.—Blood-vessels of the lungs.—Their structure and covering.—The bronchial tubes.—The pulmonary artery.—The brachial
arteries.—The lymphatics.—The nerves of the lungs.—The pleuræ.
—The mediastinum.—Professor Sweetser's ingenious description
of the lungs.

HAVING given a general view of some of the leading
features of pulmonary consumption, I now proceed to
describe the anatomy and physiology of the parts
more immediately concerned. This will aid in giving a clearer idea of the true nature of the disease, its
causes and symptoms, and of the most suitable
means for its prevention and cure.

The thorax, or chest.—The thorax, or chest, is that
cavity situated at the upper part of the trunk of the
body. It is conical in its shape, with its base below,
and apex above. It is bounded as follows : in front
by the sternum or breast bone, the sixth superior
costal cartilages, the ribs, and intercostal muscles ; on
the sides by the ribs and intercostal muscles ; and behind by the same structure, and by the spinal column,
as low down as the upper border of the last rib.
Above, it is bounded by the thoracic fasciæ, or coverings, and the first ribs, and below by the diaphragm.
This latter, which may be termed the floor of the
chest, does not lie either horizontally or flat, as may
be seen by cut No. 2, but rises into the cavity of the

chest, presenting a considerable convexity above, and a corresponding concavity below. This is its position in a relaxed state ; but when it contracts, it becomes partially flattened, so that the space above it is increased. In the diaphragm, there are apertures through which the œsophagus, larger blood-vessels, and certain nerves pass.

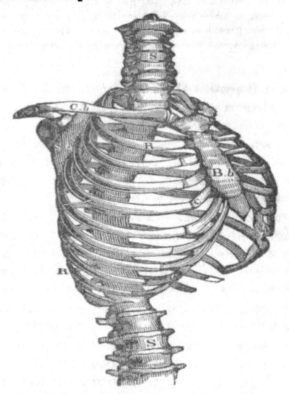

No. 1. View of the Chest.

B, b, the breast bone. R, R, the ribs. C, C, cartilages connecting the ribs with the breast bone. C, b, the collar bone. S S, the spine. S, b, the shoulder blade.

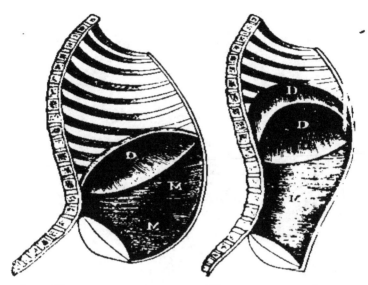

No. 2. SECTIONS OF THE CHEST AND ABDOMEN,

Showing more particularly the diaphragm. D, D, diaphragm. M, M, M, muscles of the abdomen. In the first view, the diaphragm appears as in its relaxed condition; in the second, in its contracted state. As this is drawn inward, at the same time expanding the chest, the diaphragm descends. When the air is forced outward, the diaphragm ascends.

The mechanism of respiration is beautifully illustrated by Dr. Griscom, of this city (New York), in his most valuable and instructive tracts for the people, entitled, "Uses and Abuses of Air," works which should be in the possession of every family in the land.* Figure No. 4, page 45, represents the model by which the illustration is made.

* The Uses and Abuses of air: showing its influence in sustaining life, and producing disease; with remarks on the ventilation of houses, and the best methods of securing a pure and wholesome atmosphere inside of dwellings, churches, court rooms, workshops, and buildings of all kinds. J. S. Redfield, New York.

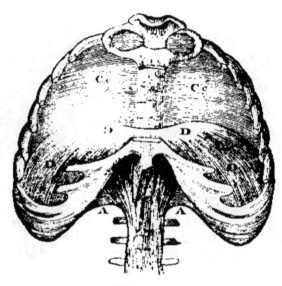

No. 3.

Front view of the chest and diaphragm; the latter relaxed. The front half of the ribs being cut away, the interior of the chest is exposed. C, c, C, c, represent the cavity of the chest empty. D, D, D, D, the diaphragm, rising high in the centre, and descending very low at the sides and behind. The white space, at its upper part, is its tendinous portion. A, A, the abdomen.

Anatomical description of the lungs, and other parts within the chest.—The trunk of the human body, which contains all its great and more important organs, except the brain, may be compared to a house two stories high. In the lower story, there are the stomach, liver, spleen, pancreas, bowels, kidneys, bladder, womb, etc. In the upper story, there are the lungs, or *lights*, heart, and large blood-vessels. The partition, or diaphragm, between these, or the floor, as we may say, of the upper story, as we have seen, crosses at the lower ribs. I cannot

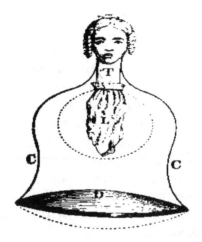

No. 4.

C, C, fig. ɑ, is a bell-shaped glass, to represent the chest. In the mouth of the glass is inserted, very tightly, a cork, T, representing the trachea, having a hole lengthwise through it. To the lower end of the cork is attached a small bladder, L, representing a lung. The lower opening of the bell is closed by a piece of sheet gum elastic, D, which fits air-tight. This answers for the *diaphragm.*

No communication can exist between the cavity of the bell and the external air, except through the hole in the cork; and any air entering through that hole can only go into the bladder. It is evident, also, that when the diaphragm is pushed into the cavity of the glass, as at D, the bladder will be flaccid and void of air; but when the diaphragm is drawn down in the situation of the dotted curve, a partial vacuum in the glass will be the consequence, which can only be supplied with air through the cork, whereby the bladder will expand to its full extent, shown by the dotted circle; and when the diaphragm is pushed up again, the air will be forced out from the bladder.

do better in giving my readers a description of the contents of the chest, than to quote the words of Dr. Erasmus Wilson, a very succinct and accurate writer on anatomy.

"*The lungs* are two conical organs, situated one on

each side of the chest, embracing the heart, and separated from each other by a membranous partition, the mediastinum. On the external or thoracic side they are convex, and correspond with the form of the cavity of the chest; internally they are concave, to receive the convexity of the heart. Superiorly they terminate in a tapering cone, which extends above the level of the first rib, and inferiorly they are broad and concave, and rest upon the convex surface of the diaphragm. Their posterior border is round and broad, the anterior sharp, and marked by one or two deep fissures, and the interior, which surrounds the base, is also sharp.

"The color of the lungs is pinkish gray, mottled, and variously marked with black. The surface is figured with irregular polygonal outlines, which represent the lobules of the organ, and the area of each of these polygonal spaces is crossed by lighter lines.

"Each lung is divided into two lobes by a long and deep fissure, which extends from the posterior surface of the upper part of the organ, downward and forward, to near the anterior angle of its base.

"In the right lung, the upper lobe is subdivided by a second fissure, which extends obliquely forward from the middle of the preceding to the anterior border of the organ, and marks off a small triangular lobe.

"The *right lung* is larger than the left, in consequence of the inclination of the heart to the left side. It is also shorter, from the great convexity of the liver, which presses the diaphragm upward upon the right side of the chest, considerably above the level of the left. It has three lobes.

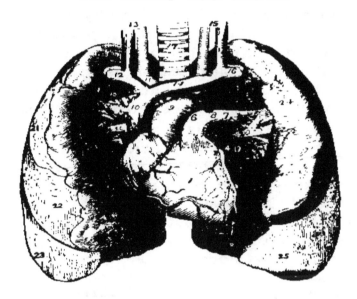

No. 5. View of the Heart and Lungs.

1. The right ventricle ; the vessels to the right of the figure are the middle coronary artery and veins ; and those to its left, the anterior coronary artery and veins. 2. The left ventricle. 3. The right auricle. 4. The left auricle. 5. The pulmonary artery. 6. The right pulmonary artery. 7. The left pulmonary artery. 8. The remains of the ductus arteriosus. 9. The arch of the aorta. 10. The superior vena cava. 11. The right arteria innominata, and in front of it, the vena innominata. 12. The right subclavian vein, and behind it, its corresponding artery. 13. The right common carotid artery and vein. 14. The left vena innominata. 15. The left carotid artery and vein. 16. The left subclavian vein and artery. 17. The trachea. 18. The right bronchus. 19. The left bronchus. 20, 20. The pulmonary veins ; 18, 20, form the root of the right lung ; and 7, 19, 20, the root of the left. 21. The superior lobe of the right lung. 22. Its middle lobe. 23. Its interior lobe. 24. The superior lobe of the left lung. 25. Its inferior lobe.

"The left lung is smaller, has but two lobes, but is longer than the right.

" Each lung is retained in its place by its *roots*, which is formed by the pulmonary artery, pulmonary veins, and bronchial tubes, together with the bronchial vessels and pulmonary plexuses of nerves. The large vessels of the root of each lung are arranged in a similar order from before, backward, on both sides, viz.,

Pulmonary veins,
Pulmonary artery,
Bronchus.

" From above downward, on the right side, this order is exactly reversed ; but on the left side the bronchus has to stoop beneath the arch of the aorta, which alters its position in the vessels. They are thus disposed on the two sides :

Right.		Left.
Bronchus,		Artery,
Artery,	——	Bronchus,
Veins.		Veins.

" *Structure of the lungs.*—The lungs are composed of the ramifications of the bronchial tubes which terminate in bronchial cells (air cells), of the ramifications of the pulmonary artery and veins, bronchial arteries and veins, lymphatics, and nerves, the whole of these structures being held together by cellular tissue, which constitutes the *parenchyma*. The parenchyma of the lungs, when examined on the surface or by means of a section, is seen to consist of small polygonal divisions, or lobules, which are connected to each other by an interlobular cellular tissue. These lobules again consist of smaller lobules, and the latter are formed by a cluster of air cells, in the parietes of which the capillaries of the pulmonary artery and pul-

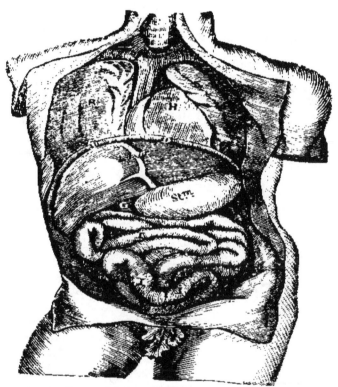

No. 6. RELATIVE POSITION OF THE LUNGS IN THE BODY.

The letters R L and L L mark the right and left lungs, with the heart H lying between them, but chiefly on the left side. V is not a very accurate representation of the large blood-vessels going to the head, neck, and superior extremities. Liv. is the liver, lying in the abdomen, or belly, and separated from the chest by the arched fleshy partition, D D, called the diaphragm, or midriff. The stomach appears on the other side, marked Stm., but both it and the liver are removed a little from their natural situation. G is the gall-bladder. I I I are the various parts of the intestinal canal, through which the food is passed on its way from the stomach, by means of what is called the PERISTALTIC or VERMICULAR motion of the bowels, one circle of fibres narrowing after another, so as to propel its contents slowly but steadily, and resembling in some degree, the condition of a worm.

3

"Each lung is retained in its place by its
is formed by the pulmonary artery, puln
and bronchial tubes, together with the
sels and pulmonary plexuses of nerves
vessels of the root of each lung are
similar order from before, backward, on

    Pulmonary veins,
    Pulmonary artery,
    Bronchus.

"From above downward, on th
order is exactly reversed; but on
bronchus has to stoop beneath the
which alters its position in the vess
disposed on the two sides:

    Right
  Bronchus,   ——
  Artery,
  Veins.

"*Structure of the lungs.—*
of the ramifications of the
minate in bronchial cell
tions of the pulmonary
arteries and veins, lym
of these structures be
sue, which constitut
chyma of the lungs
by means of a sec
gonal divisions,
each other by
lobules again
are formed b
which the c

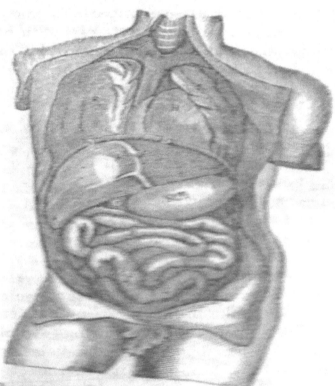

No. 6.

The letters B I and I I mean the right and left lungs...
heart H lying between them, not exactly in the ...
very accurate representation as the ...
head, neck, and superior extremities ...
abdomen, or belly, are separated from the chest in the ...
portion, D B, called the diaphragm, or midriff ...
on the other two sections, but with I and the liver ...
first ...

monary veins are distributed. * * * The walls of the air cells are so imperfect, that all the cells of any lobule communicate freely with others, while the contagious lobules are separated by the parenchyma. Dr. Horner's dissections exhibit this in a beautiful manner. See Horner's Special Anatomy, 3d edition.—G.

"*The Bronchial tubes.*—The two bronchi proceed from the bifurcation of the trachea to their corresponding lungs. The right takes its course nearly at right angle with the trachea, and enters the upper part of the right lung, while the left, longer and smaller than the right, passes obliquely beneath the arch of the aorta, and enters the lung at about the middle of its root. Upon entering the lungs they divide into two branches, and each of these divides and subdivides dichotomously to their ultimate termination in small dilated sacs, the bronchial or pulmonary cells.

" The fibro-cartilaginous rings which are observed in the trachea become incomplete and irregular in shape in the bronchi, and in the smaller bronchial tubes are lost altogether   At the termination of these tubes the fibrous and muscular coats become extremely thin, and are probably continued upon the lining mucous membrane of the air cells.

"The *pulmonary artery*, conveying the dark and impure venous blood to the lungs, terminates in capillary vessels, which form a minute network upon the parietes of the bronchial cells, and then converge to form the pulmonary veins, by which the arterial blood, purified by its passage through the capillaries, is returned to the left auricle of the heart.

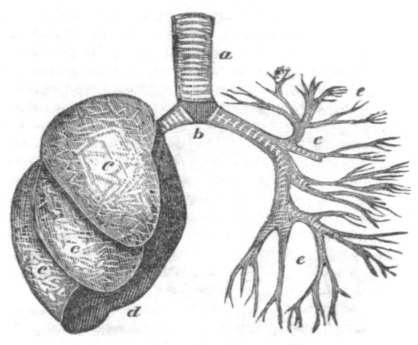

No. 7.

The letter *a* represents the trachea or wind pipe; *b*, its bifurcation or division into the two bronchial tubes; *e, e, e,* the minute ramification of the bronchi; and *c, c, c,* the right lung with its three lobes, the left having but two, to give room for the heart.

" The *Bronchial arteries*, branches of the thoracic aorta, ramify upon the bronchial tubes and in the tissue of the lungs, and supply them with nutrition, while the venous blood is returned by the bronchial veins to the vena azygos.

" The *Lymphatics*, commencing upon the surface and in the substance of the lungs, terminate in the bronchial glands. These glands, very numerous, and often of large size, are placed at the roots of the lungs, around the bronchi, and at the bifurcation of the trachea. In early life they resemble lymphatic glands in other situations; but in old age, and often in the adult, they are quite black, and filled with carbonaceous matter, and occasionally with calcareous deposits.

" The *Nerves* are derived from the pneumogastric and sympathetic. They form two plexuses—the *anterior pulmonary plexus*, situated upon the front of the root of the lungs, and composed chiefly of filaments from the great cardiac plexus; and posterior pulmonary plexus, on the posterior aspect of the root of the lungs, composed principally of branches from the pneumogastric. The branches from these plexuses follow the course of the bronchial tubes, and are distributed to the bronchial cells.

" *Pleuræ.*—Each lung is inclosed, and its structure maintained, by a serous membrane—the pleura, which invests it as far as the root, and is thence reflected upon the parietes of the chest. That portion of the membrane which is in relation with the lung is called *pleura pulmonalis*, and that in contact with the parietes *pleura costalis*. The reflected portion, besides forming the internal lining to the ribs and intercostal muscles, also covers the diaphragm and the thoracic surface of the vessels at the root of the neck.

" The pleura must be dissected from off the root of the lung, to see the vessels by which it is formed and the pulmonary plexuses.

" *Mediastinum.*—The approximation of the two reflected pleuræ in the middle line of the thorax forms a septum which divides the chest into the two pulmo-

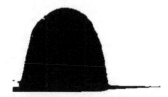

nary cavities. This is the mediastinum. The two pleuræ are not, however, in contact with each other at the middle line in the formation of the mediastinum, but leave a space between them, which contains all the viscera of the chest, with the exception of the lungs. The mediastinum is divided into the anterior, middle, and posterior.

" The *Anterior Mediastinum* is a triangular space, bounded in front by the sternum, and on each side by the pleura. It contains a quantity of loose cellular tissue, in which are found some lymphatic glands and vessels passing upward from the liver, the remains of the thymus gland, the origin of the sterno-hyoid, sterno-thyroid, and triangularis sterni-muscles, and the internal mammary vessels of the left side.

" The *Middle Mediastinum* contains the heart, inclosed in its pericardium, the ascending aorta, the superior vena cava, the bifurcation of the trachea, the pulmonary arteries, veins, and the phrenic nerves.

" The *Posterior Mediastinum* is bounded behind by the vertebral column, in front by the pericardium, and on each side by the pleura. It contains the descending aorta, the greater and lesser azygos veins, and superior intercostal vein, the thoracic duct ; the œsophagus and pneumogastric nerves, and tne great splanchnic nerves."

A very able and lucid writer, Professor Sweetser, of this city, ingeniously describes the lungs as being reared up in the following manner :

" An elastic air-tube, called the trachea or windpipe, opens into the superior portion of the throat— and consequently communicates with the mouth and posterior part of the nostrils—by a curious mechanism, in which the voice is mostly formed, called the larynx. This tube passes down the neck, enters the chest, and then forks into two divisions, called *bronchia* or *bronchi*, from a Greek word meaning the throat, one going to each lung. They then subdivide, and go on ramifying again and again, becoming smaller and smaller, and less and less elastic, until they ultimately terminate in the minute vesicles or air-cells, to which I have before alluded. These air-cells, with the air-tubes conducting to them, may be viewed as the framework of the lungs, and constitute the greater proportion of their substance. The cells, too, always contain more or less air ; it is to them that these organs owe their light and spongy character.

" The union of these little vesicles is effected through the medium of a fine membrane, denominated cellular, which, though so abundant in many other structures of the body, is here very small in quantity. Every where upon these cells, minute vessels are ramifying, to carry to them blood to be acted upon by the vital air they are continually receiving, and to convey it back again in its course to the heart, after having undergone its mysterious aerial change.

" It appears to have been a grand principle of nature, in building up the beautiful and important organs of respiration, to provide that the greatest possible quantity of blood should be brought under the influence of the greatest possible amount of air. The number of the air-cells exceed all accurate calculation. They have been estimated in man at between one and two millions, and as presenting a surface of fifteen hundred square feet. They exercise, too, as may readily be conceived, the most important agency in the breathing function, since it is during the passage of the blood over their delicate coats that the essential vital influence is wrought upon this fluid."

CHAPTER VI.

Phenomena of respiration further considered.—Its general principle explained.—Operation of the diaphragm.—The lungs and air-tubes are comparatively passive agents.—The lungs act like a pair of common bellows.—Great extent of surface in the air-cells of the lungs.—The exceeding great delicateness of this part.—The lungs are always nearly filled with air.—An important practical point.—Atmosphere within the lungs is changed gradually.—Males inhale much more than females.—Probable amount of air inhaled in twenty-four hours.—Great importance of the function of respiration.

HAVING spoken of the anatomical structure of the lungs and the adjacent parts, we are prepared to consider, in the next place, the physiology of respiration, and its effects on life.

The general principle of the operation of respiration is this: "The lungs are suspended in a cavity that is completely closed, being bounded above and around by the bony framework of the chest, the interspaces of which are filled up by the muscles and membranes, and being entirely cut off from the abdomen below by the diaphragm. Under ordinary circumstances, the lungs completely fill the cavity, their external surface, covered by the pleura, being every where in contact with the pleural lining of the chest. But the capacity of the thoracic cavity is susceptible of being greatly altered by the movements of the ribs, and by the actions of the diaphragm and abdominal muscles. When it is diminished, the lungs are compressed, and a portion of the air contained in them is expelled through the trachea. On the other hand, when it is increased, the elasticity of the air within the lungs causes them immediately to dilate so as to fill the vacuum that would otherwise exist in the thoracic cavity; and a rush of air takes place down the air-tubes and into the remotest air-cells, to equalize the density of the air they include (which has been rarefied by the dilatation of the containing cavities) with that of the surrounding atmosphere."

But the diaphragm performs the most important part in the act of inspiration. "The contraction of this muscle (see the anatomical description) changes its upper surface from the high arch that it forms, when relaxed and pushed upward by the viscera (such as the stomach, liver, spleen, bowels, etc.), to a much more level state, though it never approaches very closely to a plane, being somewhat convex even when the fullest inspiration has been taken. When thus drawn down, it presses upon the abdominal viscera, and causes them to project forward, which they are allowed to do by the relaxation of the abdominal muscles. In tranquil breathing, this action is alone nearly sufficient to produce the requisite enlargement of the thoracic cavity, the position of the ribs being very little altered. In the expiratory movement, the diaphragm is altogether passive; for being in a state of relaxation it is forced upward by the abdominal viscera, which are pressed inward by the contraction of the abdominal muscles. These last, therefore, are the

3*

main instruments of the expiratory movement, diminishing the cavity of the chest by lifting its floor at the same time they draw its bony framework into a narrower compass."

The lungs, and air-tubes conducting to them, are almost entirely passive instruments in the function of respiration. True, the contraction of the lungs when over-distended, and their dilation after extreme pressure, may be partly due to the elasticity of their structure. A moderately distended state of the lungs is that condition which seems most natural. But the fullest expansion, and the most complete contraction of which they are capable, are accomplished only by a voluntary or forcible effort.

The operation of the lungs in respiration may be compared to the action of the common bellows. When the sides of the chest are separated, and the diaphragm depressed, a vacuum takes place within this thoracic cavity, and by the pressure of the atmosphere from without, the air is made to rush through the bronchial tubes into the innumerable cavities or air-cells of the lungs. This alternate expansion and contraction of the chest and lungs go on incessantly, whether we sleep or whether we are awake, from the first moment of our existence to the very last.

The lungs are not simple hollow organs, like many others of the human body, but are composed of a sponge-like mass of cellular tissue. The trachea, or wind-pipe, as it enters the chest, is divided, as we have seen, into two branches, called bronchiæ. These pass one to each lung, and as they advance are divided and subdivided to an unlimited and inconceivable extent, terminating in the myriads of air-cells, somewhat in the same manner as the twigs of the trees terminate in leaves. It has been calculated that the number of air-cells, grouped around the extremity of each tube, is little less than 18,000, and that the total number in the lungs amount to *six hundred millions*. According to this estimate, and even admitting that it is much above the truth, it is evident that the amount of surface exposed to the atmosphere by the walls of these minute air-cells, must be many times greater than that of the exterior of the body. When we look at facts of this kind—facts, too, which cannot be at all adequately estimated or comprehended by the finite mind—we have an evidence truly, that man is most fearfully and wonderfully made.

The delicateness of the internal surface of the lungs will appear evident, when we consider their lightness or trifling weight. Notwithstanding this great amount of surface, thirty times that of the whole surface of the body, as some have reckoned, the lungs, in the largest individuals, weigh at most, only a few pounds. The lining membrane ~is so delicately and finely constructed, that it readily allows of the transmission of air through it, while the blood is retained in the appropriate vessels for that purpose.

The lungs also contain a large quantity of air. Their external surface is at all times in contact with the internal surface of the chest. The chest is formed, in a great measure, of unyielding bones and ligaments, so that it cannot change much in size after it is fully formed. Consequently, from the pressure of the atmosphere from without, the lungs must contain at all times a considerable portion of atmospheric air; enough, in short, to fill the vacuum which would otherwise be formed. It is interesting here to observe an important practical point in the function of respiration. It is easy, by well-regulated exercise, to educate the voluntary muscles of the system to almost any desirable extent. Such exercise, properly conducted, and persevered in for a sufficient length of time, must necessarily result in a greater development, size, and strength of whatever muscle is thus exercised. We know that a blacksmith strengthens his arm by the proper use of the part. The muscles of the lower extremities of sedentary persons, are very readily made larger and firmer by properly conducted pedestrian exercises. So, too, that important part of the system, the chest, one upon the development of which health so much depends, can be enlarged and invigorated to a truly wonderful extent.

The atmosphere contained within the lungs is never changed suddenly, as some might suppose. The lungs never empty themselves at any one time. A small portion only, comparatively, is received at each inspiration, and at each expiration a corresponding portion is thrown off. An ordinary inspiration is reckoned at from one to two pints, while the average capacity of the lungs, when the chest is fully expanded, is estimated at about twelve pints. There would thus be left in the lungs, after an ordinary expiration, the remaining ten or eleven pints of air, which serve to keep the air-cells continually distended. Public singers and speakers, and such as habitually use their lungs to a greater than ordinary degree, especially if this be practiced in the open air, it is ascertained may take in at a single inspiration from five to seven pints at a time. By this wonderful power of adaptation, which these delicate structures possess, some very interesting and remarkable effects in vocal and instrumental music may be performed.

There appears to be a great difference between the capacity of the lungs for air, between males and females. Thus Mr. Thackrah (as quoted by Dr. Combe) mentions that men can exhale, at one effort, from six to ten pints of air ; whereas, in women the average is only from two to four pints. In ten females, about eighteen and-a-half years of age, belonging to a flax-mill, and who were laboring under no disease, Mr. Thackrah found the average to be only three and one-half pints, while in young men of the same age, it amounted to six pints.

Thus it appears that physiologists vary in their estimates as to the amount of air inhaled and exhaled at each respiration. It is difficult to arrive at the exact truth in matters of this kind, nor is this strictly necessary for practical purposes.

At the rate of from one to two pints at each inspiration, an almost incredible amount of air is received into the lungs every twenty-four hours. The average number of respirations is about eighteen per minute. Consequently, the number for one hour is one thousand and eighty ; in twenty-four hours, twenty-five thousand nine hundred and twenty. Allowing eighteen pints of air—the lowest estimate—to be inhaled every minute, there would be upward of *fifty hogsheads* inhaled each twenty-four hours. The largeness of this amount must serve to impress every one with the importance of paying particular attention to the quality of this life-giving fluid, which is daily and hourly received into these delicate structures of the system, and on the proper state of which life and health so much depend.

Must it not be always an important consideration whether this air be pure or impure? in other words, whether good or bad? We may subsist for days, and even weeks, without food and drink, but if respiration be cut short for *three minutes only*, death is the inevitable result.

CHAPTER VII.

Circulation of the blood.—The blood of two kinds.—The heart, arteries, and veins.—Action of the heart described.—The two rounds of circulation.—The arterial blood and the venous.—The never-ceasing action of the heart.—Amount of blood passing through the heart, and to the lungs, per hour.—Amount of air necessary to purify it.—Practical deductions from the foregoing facts.

THE nature and importance of the function of respiration will become still more apparent by considering, in this connection, the circulation of the blood.

The blood, which circulates every where throughout the living body, is of two kinds: the one dark, impure, venous blood ; the other red, pure, or arterialized blood. The latter, alone, is capable of supporting life.

The heart—with its accompaniments, the arteries and veins—is the great organ by which the circulation of the blood is effected. It is a muscular organ, having somewhat the shape of an inverted cone, lying in the lower part of the thoracic cavity, between the two folds of the pleura, which form the central partition of the chest. (See cut No. 8.) It lies partly on the middle line, and partly on the left side of the chest. Strictly speaking, it is a double organ, with two corresponding halves. Each half is also divided into an upper and lower cavity, the upper being called auricles, and the lower ventricles. The right auricle receives the dark blood coming in the veins from all

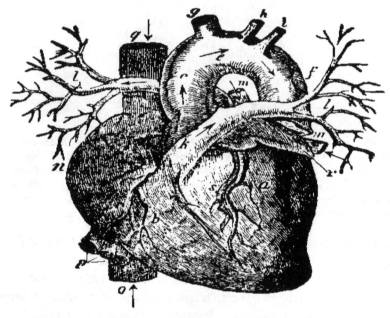

No. 8.   The Heart.

a, the left ventricle; *b*, the right ventricle: *c, e, f*, the aorta, the great artery that goes off from the left ventricle; *g, k, i*, the arteries that are sent from the arch of the aorta; *k*, the pulmonary artery, that goes from the right ventricle to the lungs; *l, l*, branches of the pulmonary artery, going to the two sides of the lungs; *m, m*, the pulmonary veins, which bring the blood back from the lungs to the left side of the heart; *n*, the right auricle; *o*, the ascending vena cava; *q*, the descending; these two meet, and by their union form the right auricle; *p*, the veins from the liver, spleen, and bowels; *s*, the left coronary artery, one of the arteries which nourish the heart.

parts of the body. From this it is sent through a valve into the right ventricle; from the right ventricle the blood is sent through a vessel which divides itself into two branches, one of which goes to each lung. These are called pulmonary arteries, although they

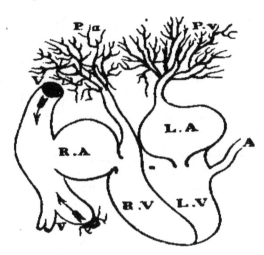

No. 9. RELATIVE POSITION AND MODE OF COMMUNICATION BETWEEN THE CAVITIES OF THE HEART.

Two large veins, V, V—one descending from the head and upper extremities, the other ascending from the lower extremities, abdomen, and other parts—receive all the impure blood from the body, and unite together near the right auricle (R, A). They pour their joint currents into that chamber, and distend it. When filled, it contracts upon its contents, and forces the fluid into the right ventricle (R, V). This, when filled, contracts, and drives the blood into the pulmonary artery (P. *a*), which carries it all to the two lungs, dividing it between them, through appropriate branches, and distributing it, in minute particles, over the surface of the pulmonary air cells. Its color is yet of a dark purple; but immediately, as it is distributed through the lungs, and is acted upon by the air in the cells, its color changes, and becomes a bright vermilion, or scarlet. This change having been effected, it is again collected from the lungs by means of another set of blood-vessels, called pulmonary veins (P, v.) which convey it away from the lungs, and carry it back to the heart, where, the vessels from each lung uniting, it is emptied into the *left* auricle (L, A). From this it is thrown into the left ventricle (L, V). From this cavity arises the main artery of the body, the *aorta* (A); and through this great tube the purified blood is sent, to be distributed all over the body, visiting every fibre and atom for their sustenance and growth.

carry dark or venous blood. "In the innumerable branches of this artery, expanding themselves throughout the substance of the lungs, the dark blood is subjected to the contact of the air inhaled in breathing; and a change in the composition, both of the blood and the inhaled air, takes place, in consequence of which the former is found to have reassumed its florid or arterial hue, and to have regained its power of supporting life." The blood then enters the myriads of minute venous ramifications, which gradually coalesce into larger branches, and at last terminate in four large trunks, two from each lung, and empty themselves into the left auricle, from which the blood is thrown into the left ventricle, and from this through the great aorta, which divides itself again into myriads of arteries, greater and smaller, through which the purified or arterial blood is distributed to every part of the body, however minute.

Thus, it will be seen, there are in the living body two distinct circulations, each carried on by its own system of vessels. First, the impure blood comes from every part of the body to the right side of the heart. It is sent thence to the lungs to be purified. It returns to the left side of the heart, and is sent from thence throughout the whole body for the maintenance of life. Neither the crude blood, which is formed from the food in the living laboratory, nor the dark venous blood, can afford any nourishment to the living body until having been subjected to the purifying influence of the atmosphere in the lungs. Venous blood in the arteries is indeed positively poisonous. The heart, as every one knows, acts by pulsations. It is composed of an involuntary muscle, as we say. It goes on both by night and by day, both when we sleep and when we wake, throughout our whole life. It is an organ over which we have no direct or voluntary control.

It is a beautiful phenomenon of nature that the pulsations of the heart, and the movements of the chest and lungs, harmonize with each other, or have a relation which in health is always maintained. The office of respiration is to induce a constant supply of pure air into the lungs, by which the blood becomes arterialized or purified.

There is an average of four pulsations of the heart to one respiration. The average number of respirations is about eighteen per minute. In infancy it is more, about twenty-five per minute. In old age it is less, about sixteen per minute ; but at whatever age, the relation between the respirations of the lungs, and the pulsations of the heart, remain the same. When there are seventy-two pulsations of the heart per minute, as may be ascertained by the pulse at the wrist, there are one fourth as many respirations, namely, eighteen in the same period of time.

The amount of blood sent to the lungs at each pulsation of the heart, in an adult individual of average weight, may be reckoned at about two ounces. According to this estimate, then, more than *twenty-five hogsheads* of blood are sent through the heart, and to the lungs, every day of the individual's life, and to purify this blood, more than twice the amount of air must be inhaled !

When, therefore, we consider the important relations that exist between respiration and circulation, and the most intimate dependence of life at all times on these functions, numerous practical inferences are suggested to the mind.   Thus it will be apparent, that the *quality* of the air breathed must be ever an important consideration in regard to health.   So, too, the quality of the blood which is to be changed constantly by the wonderful, nay, mysterious, action of the air upon it!   What food shall we eat?   What air shall we breathe?   What exercise, mental and physical, shall we take?   These are important questions, and such as concern every individual, in proportion as health is the best of all earthly gifts.   These considerations will be entered into more in detail in another part of the work.

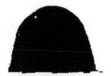

CHAPTER VIII.

Tubercles, the foundation of true pulmonary consumption.—Meaning
of the word tubercle.—Character of tubercles.—Tuberculous deposits may occur in nearly every part of the body.—Tables showing
their relative frequency in the different organs and parts.—Dr.
Good's remarks on the subject.—Tubercles may probably remain
many years in the system without endangering life.—They ordinarily increase in number and size, and have a greater tendency
to inflame and maturate as years advance.—Process of maturation.—Can tuberculous disease be cured?—Opinions of various
authors on the subject.—Animals often have tubercles.—How
caused.—The milch cows of Paris.—Practical inferences from the
foregoing facts.

TUBERCLE being considered the foundation or germ
of true consumption, this abnormal structure or
condition of the living parts will now be considered.

The word tubercle is derived from the Latin term,
tuberculum, which signifies an excrescence, tumor, or
swelling of some part of the living body. In pathological anatomy, the term is applied to a diseased product, or species of degeneration, which is composed of
"an opaque matter, of a pale yellow color," resembling
cheese in its color and consistence. They vary much
in size, from that of a pin-head up to the size of an
orange. When, however, they have become large,
it is supposed that many must have coalesced or come
together. They are probably always small at first,
but as they grow larger, many become amalgamated
into one. They are at first, perhaps, always more

grayish and semi-transparent than opaque and yellow. It is when they have increased in size and number, and when many have grown into one, that they take on this latter character.

"When tubercles are few," says Dr. Elliotson, " they seldom exceed the size of an almond each, but the masses produced by their aggregation, may be very large." The whole of a lobe of the lung may become converted into a solid tubercular mass, and it is said, indeed, that a whole lung has, in certain cases, become thus affected.

Tubercles may occur in almost any part of the body. Indeed no part, with the exception of the bones and the external skin, may be said to be wholly exempt from a liability to them. According to a table quoted by Sir James Clark, the result of fifty careful post-mortem examinations of children, made with the view of determining the relative frequency of tubercles in different organs, was as follows:

Bronchial glands (glands of the wind-pipe),....	49 times.
Lungs,................................	38 "
Cervical glands (glands of the neck),..........	26 "
Mesenteric glands (in the abdomen),.........	25 "
Spleen,................................	20 "
Pleura (lining membrane of the chest),........	17 "
Liver,................................	14 "
Small intestines,..........................	12 "
Peritoneum (surrounding membrane of the intestines),.............	9 "
Large intestines,........	9 "
Brain,................................	5 "
Cerebellum,............................	3 "
Membranes of the brain,...................	3 "

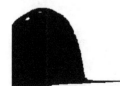

Pericardium (covering membrane of the heart),	0	times.
Kidneys,................................	2	"
Stomach,.................................	1	"
Pancreas,................................	1	"
Vertebræ, radius, tibia (bones of the spine, forearm, and leg),...........................	1	"

A table of Louis, showing the relative frequency of tubercles in the different organs, referring to persons above the age of fifteen who died of consumption, is as follows :

Tubercles in the	small	intestines,..........	1 case in	3
"	"	large,.................	1 "	9
"	"	mesenteric glands,.......	1 "	4
"	"	cervical,...............	1 "	10
"	"	lumber glands,..........	1 "	12
"	"	spleen,................	1 "	14
"	"	prostate,..............	1 "	13
"	"	ovaries,...............	1 "	20
"	"	kidneys,...............	1 "	40

These persons having all died of consumptions, had, of course, tubercles in the lungs, as well as in the other organs mentioned.

Dr. Good gives similar testimony to the above in regard to tubercles. He observes : " There is not an organ of the body but is capable, as well in its substance as its parenchyma (covering), of producing tubercles of some kind or other ; and occasionally of almost every kind at the same time ; for Bonet, Boerhaave and De Haen, as well as innumerable writers in our own day, have given striking examples of clusters of cystic tubers, or enlarged tubercles, of every diversity of size, existing both in the abdomen and in the thorax

(chest), formed in the interior of their respective viscera, or issuing from the surface of their serous membranes, some of which are filled with a limpid fluid,
others with a gelatinous, a mucous, or a puriform, and
others again with a cheesy, pulpy, or steatomatous
mass."

It is supposed, although it cannot be proved positively, that tubercles may remain many years in an
uninflamed or quiescent state ; and this must depend
much upon the general habits of the individual. Bad
habits, bad air, bad food, and bad influences generally,
develop them often to a fearful extent.

Ordinarily, when tubercles have been once formed,
they go on augmenting in size more or less rapidly,
according to the habits of the individual, the climate
in which he lives, and all the varying influences which
go to operate on the health, until they are converted
at last into a fluid mass, resembling common pus.
This may be said to resemble unstrained whey, and is
sometimes stained with blood, or a black matter formed
in the lungs.   As this stage of maturation or softening
goes on, the fluid mass finds its way into the air passages, and is expelled from the lungs day by day, by
expectoration, leaving an ulcerous excavation or cavern, as some call it, in the lungs.   In some cases this
process of ulceration appears to remain nearly station-
ary for an indefinite time, until at last the individual
sinks under it.

Is tuberculous disease curable ?   It has been regarded by many that tuberculous diseases of the lungs
are never cured.   These morbid productions are
found in the youngest children, even in the unborn

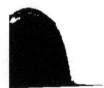

infant; and from this up to the octogenarian, and how much older we do not know. But that tubercles can never be cured is not yet proved. The world generally has poor notions of what it is possible to do by a combination of good general circumstances, in the curing of these worst forms of disease. If we take a number of dirty children—those of the lowest and most unhealthy and miserable class in any of our great cities, and remove them to a good air, keep them clean, give them good food, and, in short, bring them up in accordance with the principles of physiological science, we find that most of them will get along remarkably well, better than children ordinarily do whose parents are in good circumstances. Such things have been done over and over again.

I visited two years since the Hamburgh Redemption Institute, as it is called in this country, an institution in which has been received for some twenty years the most miserable of the children of the city of Hamburgh; and the worthy founder of this charity informed me that they were never sick. It is situated a few miles in the country, in a very pleasant healthy place. Every thing in regard to sleeping, eating, drinking, occupation, amusements, etc., is carried on with the utmost regularity. Good food is furnished, but of the plainest kinds. I asked if the children had any tea, coffee, beer, or like drinks; I was answered by the worthy pastor, " No, they have only water-gruel or milk. We regard this much more healthful, and it is not too much to say that our children never become sick." So much for temperance, regularity, healthful employment of mind and body, and the in-

4

fluence of a rational religion daily carried out, and this too among the most dirty, miserable, degraded, and most badly born children of the city of Hamburgh, in Germany. Taking a hint from this pattern insti-tution, what might not people accomplish with all the health, prosperity and abundance of these United States? People ought no more to become sick than drunk.

The following extract from Dr. Dunglison, of Phila-delphia, will give the reader an idea of the prevailing opinions, concerning this subject, among medical men.

"It has been a prevalent opinion, that when once a cavern has formed in the lungs, it is incapable of cicatrization; and Dr. Chapman, of Philadelphia, has pronounced the opposite opinion to be an illusion. One of the most distinguished of modern pathologists, M. Louis, has affirmed that, in the numerous dissec-tions which he has made, he has never met with a single example. His negative experience has, how-ever, been controverted by the positive observation of others. The author has met with several instances, in which this change was unequivocally accomplish-ed; and the details of the case of an eminent medical practitioner in this city, Dr. Parrish, have been pub-lished, in whose lungs there were marked evidences of cicatrization. This probability occurred after he had long suffered under symptoms of phthisis, and ex-posed himself to a regimen as will be mentioned here-after. M. Boudet affirmed, before the *Academie Royale des Sciences*, of Paris, that, in 197 cases taken indiscriminately, he found ten examples of cavern completely cicatrized, without any trace of recent tubercles ; and eight examples of complete, or partial cure of cavern, coinciding with recent tubercles ; and he concludes, that recovery is possible at any period of pulmonary consumption. His researches would seem to show, that tubercles of the lungs are common when no suspicion is entertained of their existence. Of the 197 persons who died in the hospitals of various diseases, or were killed suddenly by accidents, he detected tubercles in the lungs of one—a child under two years of age ; from this age, to that of fifteen, tubercles were present in three fourths of the cases ; and in those between fifteen and seventy-six, no fewer than six sevenths of the bodies exhibited the tubercular deposits in the lungs. These results are explained by M. Boudet, by the facility with which tubercles undergo a change in their intimate constitution, by which they become not incompatible with a state of health. These modes of cure, according to him, consist of sequestration, induration, absorption, and elimination, which supervene spontaneously. Observers are every day discovering appearances, or dissections, which can only be referred to the existence of tubercular deposits at a former period. Of seventy-three bodies examined by Dr. H. Bennett, between November, 1844, and April, 1845, he found puckerings, or concretions, in twenty-eight ; in twelve of these, indurations alone existed ; and in sixteen, calcareous concretions were also present. In 100 bodies examined by M. Rogee, at La Salpetriere, these lesions were discovered in fifty-one, or more than one half. M. Boudet also states, that of 135 bodies examined by him, he found them in 116, or in about four fifths of the whole number. Dr. Hughes arrives at the startling conclusion, from his own observations, and those of MM. Rogee and Boudet, that the spontaneous cure of tubercle has occurred in from one third to one half of all who die after forty. ' So deeply rooted, however,' he adds, ' is the opinion of the necessarily fatal nature of this disease, that, simply because recovery has taken place in certain cases, medical men have rather mistrusted their own diagnosis,' than ventured to oppose a dogma of universal belief."

Dr. Cullen, who was a practitioner of great celebrity and experience in the last century, regarded that the prospect for recovery in consumption is for the most part unfavorable ; and that of those affected with it, the greater number die. " But there are always," says he, " many of them who recover entirely, after having been in very unpromising circumstances." He published the following aphorisms as the result of his observations:

" 1. A consumption arising from pulmonary hæmorrhage is more frequently recovered than when arising from tubercles.

" 2. A pulmonary hæmorrhage not only is not always followed by a consumption, but even when followed by an ulceration, this latter is sometimes attended with little of hectic, and frequently admits of being soon healed. Even when the hæmorrhage and ulceration have appeared to be repeated, there are instances of persons recovering entirely, after several such repetitions.

" 3. A consumption arising from a suppuration in

consequence of inflammation of the lungs, is that which most rarely occurs in this climate (Ireland) ; and a consumption does not always follow such suppuration, when the abscess formed soon breaks and discharges a laudable (healthy) pus. But if the abscess continue long shut up, and till after a considerable degree of hectic has been formed, a consumption is then produced, equally dangerous as that from other causes.

" 4. A consumption from tubercles has, I think, been recovered ; but it is of all others the most dangerous ; and when arising from an hereditary taint, is almost certainly fatal.

" 5. The danger of a consumption, from whatever cause it may have arisen, is most certainly to be judged of by the degree to which the hectic and its consequences have arrived. From a certain degree of emaciation, debility, profuse sweating, and diarrhœa no person recovers.

" 6. A mania coming on, has been found to remove all the symptoms, and sometimes has entirely cured the disease ; but, in other cases, upon the going off of the mania the consumption has recurred, and proved fatal.

" 7. Pregnancy has often retarded the progress of consumption ; but commonly it is only till after delivery, when the symptoms of the disease return with violence, and soon prove fatal."

Various authors have given accounts of cases in which it was found after death that there were cicatrizations or scars in the substance of the pulmonary tissue, proving to a most positive demonstration that ulceration had at some period existed. Every medical man, too, who has had a few years' experience in treating the disease, must have found cases in which all the more prominent symptoms existed, and in which the individuals have recovered, even contrary to his most sanguine expectations.

Considering, then, how alarming the ravages of consumption are becoming in the United States, and at the same time the pernicious nature of the physiological and hygienic habits of the community generally, may we not confidently hope that by the promulgation of correct principles of health much may yet be done in staying the course of this most fearful disease. Beyond a doubt many might be saved who, under the existing modes of hygiene and medical treatment, now sink prematurely with tubercular disease. These considerations will be entered upon in another part of the work.

Unhealthy animals also are subject to tubercles.— The morbid productions of which we have been speaking, are not peculiar to the human species. In menageries, where animals are kept in a state which is certainly very far removed from being the natural one, the animals are often affected with a cough, and the other symptoms of pulmonary consumption. Their lungs, too, are often found after death to have become ulcerous, and are filled with tubercles. The monkey family, it is said, too, when removed from their climate to colder regions, and are at the same time kept in a confined and unnatural state, frequently die of tubercular disease. The lungs of the domestic animals, as the horse, ox, cow, sheep, hog, rabbit, and other of the mammalia, are also frequently to be found tuberculous.

It is said a dog, however, is rarely affected with them. Tubercles have also been found in the bodies of domestic birds, as the turkey, fowl, etc. According to M. Andral, most of the animals in which tubercles are found to exist, are either transported from a hot to a cold climate, where they are deprived of their liberty and exercise, as in the instance of monkeys and parrots ; or else confined in damp situations, without the light of the sun, and almost without air, as cows, pigs, and house rabbits ; or exposed to constant alternations of heat and cold, or to constrained and violent exercise, as in the case of the horse.

"All the milch cows in Paris, and no doubt elsewhere," says Sir James Clark, "become tuberculous after a certain period of confinement. I have been informed that for some time after the disease has commenced, the quantity of milk obtained is greater than before, and that their flesh is more esteemed by the unsuspecting epicure than that of the healthy animal. A circumstance of the same kind is mentioned by Aristotle, who observed tubercles in the pig, the ox, and the ass ; in regard to strumous pigs, he says that when the disease (*grandines*) exists in a slight degree, the flesh is sweeter."

When we thus learn how easily tubercles may be generated in animals by taking them out of their own climate, and by placing them in unnatural and unhealthful conditions, how deep and lasting should the impression be made upon our minds, that disease is, as a general fact, a thing of man's own begetting ; that the race is, as a whole, accountable for the diseases with which it is afflicted !

CHAPTER X.

The different forms of consumption —That of infants and children.—
In them the symptoms are usually more strongly marked than in
adults.—There may also be great obscurity of the disease.—Cases
in point.—Consumption of adults.—The latent form.—The chronic.
—Acute, rapid, or quick consumption.—This may result from the
latent form.—It is oftenest seen in young females.—No two cases
of consumption in all respects alike.

Consumption of infants and children.—Formerly,
more than latterly, tuberculous disease was supposed
to be an infrequent cause of death in infancy and
childhood.　But since pathological anatomy has been
studied with greater care, infants and children have
been found to be much more subject to scrofulous disease than was formerly imagined.　Dr. Guersent, of
Paris, one of the physicians to the *Hospital des Enfans
Malades*—an institution appropriated to the treatment
of patients between the ages of one and sixteen years
—states, as the result of his observations, that five
sixths of those who died in that establishment are
more or less tuberculous.

The symptoms of consumption in cases of children
are less strongly marked than in adults; and it is to
this fact that we must attribute the former belief,
that tuberculous disease can rarely happen in infants.
The hectic fever, in children, is less perfectly
formed than in adults.　The perspirations are less
copious, and the cough is of a different character,

and much less prominent than that which accompanies consumption in persons of mature age. The cough occurs frequently in paroxysms, resembling those of pertussis, or hooping-cough. In many cases, especially in young children, there is little or no expectoration, unless, perhaps, at a late period of the disease; the matter, too, is probably often swallowed, so that we have no visible signs whatever of its existence. It will be seen from the description, that the consumption of infants and children must sometimes be very difficult of detection; but Sir James Clark regards that this will not usually be the case if we attend to the other symptoms. He observes: " The tuberculous aspect of the child, the rapid pulse and breathing, the frequent cough, and the gradually increasing emaciation commonly afford sufficient evidence of its nature. Consumption in children is often preceded or accompanied by considerable derangement of the digestive organs: the abdomen is tumid, the bowels are irregular, at one time constipated, and affected by diarrhœa at another; the evacuations in either case are generally of a pale, unnatural color. This deranged state of the functions of the abdominal viscera has led to the belief that the mesenteric glands are the chief seat of tuberculous disease; whereas, in reality, the bronchial glands and lungs are most commonly affected. It is true that the mesenteric glands become tuberculous more frequently in infancy and childhood than at a later period of life, but by no means so generally, nor to such an extent, as is supposed."

But there must every now and then cases occur, I think, in which it will be very difficult, nay, impossible to

4*

ascertain whether real consumption exists. While, on the one hand, cases occur which pass for consumption, there yet being no real disease of the lungs, the cough being only a symptom of other and fatal disease, there are, on the other, cases where the lungs are deeply and fatally diseased, and yet, at the same time, none of the plain, characteristic, and decided symptoms of the disease, such as are usually found, appear. Every practitioner who has had some years of experience in these matters, and who has watched studiously the manifestations of pulmonary disease, must have encountered cases in which he has found himself greatly mistaken in the opinions he has formed of the individual case. Thus, he will at one time believe that he can cure a case without difficulty, but on trial it grows worse and worse, till at last the patient passes into a rapid emaciation and death. But in other cases, which unfortunately happen far less often, he will believe that the individual must inevitably sink, and yet, after some months, or, perhaps, years, he is surprised to learn that his patient has recovered. I repeat, every one who has had any considerable experience in the treatment of pulmonary diseases, must acknowledge frankly to himself that he has been not unfrequently thus misled in his opinions. There are many cases of the kind in the records of medicine.

The late and talented Dr. Dewees, of Philadelphia, whose great experience as well as his candor, and his true love of the profession, make his opinions valuable on the subject, gives, in his Practice of Physic, published in Philadelphia the following cases. He observes :

"Drs Physic, Otto, and myself attended a young lady of this city, and in the course of the disease which destroyed her, there was not a single symptom that betrayed there was the slightest mischief working in the lungs ; there was neither cough, difficulty of breathing, hectic fever, nor purulent expectoration, which Pinel makes constitute phthisis ; there was marasmus, but it was not excessive. On opening the body, the lungs alone were found diseased. In another instance, Dr. Chapman and myself attended a boy, eight or nine years old, whose disease appeared to be located in the abdomen—in this part he appeared to suffer excruciating agony, which powerful doses of laudanum would scarcely abate ; and this continued to the last moment of his existence. Indeed, we may look upon Bayle's 38th and 39th cases, as being cases without the pathognomonic signs of phthisis.

"On opening the body, none of the abdominal viscera were at all diseased ; the lungs alone were the seat of the disorder. They contained very large quantities of the most offensive pus I ever remember to have encountered ; yet in this case there was not a solitary symptom to direct attention to the chest. Bayle has, therefore, said correctly, that the artificial 'character of phthisis is not applicable to all its degrees, or to all cases, and that the " essential" would not be sufficient to know it by during life.' In fact, we have no pathognomonic symptoms of phthisis— the knife alone reveals its existence with absolute certainty. * * We might, with much safety, include stethoscope ; but this instrument is so little understood in this country, and employed so rarely, that we hardly dare at this time consider it as a discriminating means, though it is absolutely one of great certainty."

It is but just to the public, to those for whom I write, that I should make known these difficulties—these uncertainties of the healing art. People have too often a blind confidence in physicians, and would appear to suppose them to know far more than it is possible for mortal mind to comprehend. There is a habit, too, among medical men—by far too common—of putting on an air of knowledge and wisdom and infallibility which they never possessed, and which indeed none *can* ever possess. As a consequence of such medical habits, the profession become narrow and bigoted in intellect, and the people have in the end less confidence in them than would be the case if they passed for what they are worth, and no more. In this, as in all other things, the old maxim of honesty holds good.

Consumption of adults.—Writers speak of a number of varieties of consumption in grown persons, such as the *latent*, the *slow* or *chronic*, and the *acute, rapid* or *quick* consumption. The peculiarities of each of these I will briefly enumerate.

Latent consumption.—Of 112 cases recorded by M. Louis, eight were latent, a smaller proportion, Dr. Clark is inclined to believe, than generally occurs from the history of these cases, and on attentive and minute examination of the lungs after death, not only of the lungs but of all the other organs. M. Louis entertained no doubt of the existence of tubercles during a period, varying from six months to two years in different cases, previous to their presence being indicated by coughing and the most common local symptoms. Dr. Clark is also of opinion—indeed, he says that he has obtained satisfactory evidence, that in some cases tuberculous disease nad commenced in the lungs from one to two years, or longer, before it was properly attended to, or its nature understood.

Middle life is supposed to be most liable to this variety of consumption, but no age is probably exempt from it.

In this variety of the disease, the tuberculous product may exist evidently for a considerable time, longer or shorter, and to a considerable extent, without occasioning any of those more common and prominent symptoms of consumption which we ordinarily see, such as cough, expectoration, or hæmorrhage, yet it goes on as surely, although not so rapidly, effecting its work of destruction as if these symptoms existed.

In some of these cases there may be observed a hectic feverishness, night sweats, wasting of the flesh, diarrhœa, etc., without any local indications of the pulmonary disease.

In other cases, the malady is more insidious in its nature, and each of the constitutional and local symptoms are either not present, or in a degree so slight as to be very difficult to determine. At length the individual passes suddenly into a very rapid consumption, that soon destroys his life.

The chronic form.—The symptoms of chronic consumption are often obscure, especially in its earlier stages; yet they are more prominent and easily distinguished than in the so-called latent form. All cases of consumption are in some sense chronic, but the term is used to designate such as are more slow in their progress, and liable to interruption from other causes. This form of the disease may continue for several years in its course, subject, however, to considerable pauses and variations. M. Louis has given cases of ten, twelve, fourteen, and twenty years' duration; and it has been known to have lasted even forty years.

Older persons, more than younger, are subject to chronic consumption. It is quite apt to occur even after the fortieth year. The individual gradually finds himself growing languid, and less capable of exertion than formerly. He has now and then a slight cough, but it is, however, scarcely sufficient to attract attention. He may have little or no feverishness, and the appetite, on the whole, may be very good. At times, again, the disease assumes a more serious aspect. In the more inclement seasons of the year, he perhaps takes a cold in the head, which results in cough of considerable severity, sometimes, indeed, very severe, and which is attended by fever and copious expectoration. These attacks may appear often to threaten life seriously, and yet the individual recovers from them, and thus goes on from year to year with little apparent advancement of the disease. Such patients are often subject to dyspepsy, and sometimes to diarrhœa; hence both the patient and his friends are apt to attribute his complaint to a fault of the stomach and digestive organs. Such patients grow pale and thin; and although they may eat heartily generally, and the appetite be remarkably good, they do not get flesh.

Indeed, the more they eat the less flesh they appear to have. They may be able to transact their ordinary avocations, whether physical or mental, but with less alacrity than usual. They are *short winded*, as horsemen say, and can bear but little fatigue, especially in ascending hills or mountains. They are, however, compelled to be scrupulously mindful of their health, and are not unfrequently ranked among that unhappy class of individuals who are supposed to be more indolent than sick. They are valetudinarians—neither on the sick list, nor are they by any means well

"The aggravations and pauses in chronic consumption are more or less frequent and distinct in different cases; the former being far more common in the cold, the latter in the summer, months. Hence the sufferer will often appear to be fast approaching the goal of his being; his fate is even pronounced, when, unexpectedly to all, the threatening symptoms abate, his health rapidly grows better, and thus, for the time being, he disproves the prediction both of physician and friends."

This form of consumption may at any time run into the acute; and I think it will be found generally to end in what may be termed the acute attack, or, perhaps, more correctly, the acute exacerbation of the disease.

Acute, rapid, or quick consumption.—The duration of consumption is more commonly from nine to thirty months; but, in what is popularly termed quick consumption, the disease frequently runs its course in two or three months, and occasionally less. Persons have died often in a single month from the disease. This form of tuberculous pulmonary affection, has been aptly termed *"galloping"* consumption. The disease is more apt to take on this rapid form when developed by some other disease, as a fever, small-pox, scarletina, measles, and the like. A common inflammation of the lungs, where tubercles have been supposed to exist, not unfrequently ends in acute consumption. The inflammation, it is supposed, serves to bring into action the tuberculous disease.

Acute consumption is evidently often only the result of the latent form ; and exposure to cold, inflammation of the lungs, over-exertion, an attack of catarrh, or hæmorrhage from the lungs, serves to develop the malady, which, although unperceived, has been for a long time performing its silent work. In such cases, we may suppose, that when the tuberculous deposit is thus brought into vigorous action, or, in other words, an active state of disease, consumption proceeds in its course with the most fearful rapidity. This form of consumption is most frequent in young persons, particularly young females, and oftener with those who inherit the scrofulous or tuberculous habit. It happens more commonly in the earlier periods of puberty, and especially with those in whom the menstrual function becomes deranged. "Such individuals seem as frail as the leaves of autumn, and fall almost as readily. They are often peacefully sinking into the arms of death before their danger is even suspected."

In the varieties of pulmonary consumption, we have—

1. That which affects infants and children, an ob-

more forms of the disease, and one which it is sometimes impossible to detect.

In actute, we observe three varieties:

1. That which is latent, or unsuspected, and which is often very difficult, and sometimes impossible to determine.

2. The chronic variety, in which the symptoms are more marked and distinct in character, and which may pass into the acute attack, or be merged into one.

3. The acute variety, which happens oftenest in young persons, especially young females, runs its course frequently with great rapidity, causing death in one, two, or three months; but which may also precede or follow the latent and chronic varieties of the disease.

Thus I have explained briefly of the different varieties of forms of pulmonary consumption. It must be remembered, however, that we can find no two cases which are in all particulars exactly alike; often, too, one form of the disease blends with another. Latent consumption may become active, and the chronic rapidly may suddenly become acute. On the other hand, too, the acute variety may pass off and turn into the chronic or latent; and thus the rapid really fatal into the mild or acute. The distinction made, may, however, still somewhat toward the guiding a knowledge of the disease.

CHAPTER XI.

Symptoms of consumption.—Hæmorrhage from the lungs.—Bronchitis.—Cough.—Hooping cough.—Spasmodic cough.—Nervous or hysterical cough.—Short, dry, or hacking cough.—Aphonic cough.—Stridulous, barking, wheezing, or whistling cough.—Loose cough.—Hoarse, loud, dry, forcible cough—Asthmatic cough.—Cough sometimes occurs in pregnancy.—Cough generally one of earliest symptoms of consumption.—Dyspnoea, or difficult breathing.—The expectoration.—Dr. Cullen's rules for distinguishing pus.—Dr. Marshall Hall's observations on expectoration.

Hæmoptysis or hæmorrhage from the lungs.—Pulmonary hæmorrhage is a frequent symptom attending consumption, although not always present. I regard it as being, in the majority of cases where it occurs, a symptom of less importance and less danger than is generally supposed. It, however, always indicates a wrong state of things in the general health, and, as such, merits, in every case, careful consideration. In some cases it is one of the most fatal of all affections of the pulmonary organs. The subject being connected with a great variety of circumstances, I have devoted a separate chapter to the consideration of its nature, causes, and effects, and the means of prevention and treatment to be employed. To these the reader is referred to another part of the work.

Bronchitis.—Bronchitis, or inflammation of the bronchial tubes often comes as a prelude to this dis-

ea se. It s indeed to be reckoned as one of its exciting
ca ises, a though we have no positive proof that actual
tubercles are ever thus brought into existence. But
this affection, as well also as chronic sore throat, will
be more fully considered in another place.

Cough.—This is a spasmodic action, more or less
violent, of the parts composing the throat and the
lungs and chest; a full inspiration of air is taken into
the lungs, then the glottis is closed pretty firmly, and
in inspiration the air forced suddenly out, and with it
frequently mucous or other matters which had irritated the air passages. Cough is generally, though
not always, one of the normal efforts of nature to
expel from the throat and lungs, more especially the
latter, things which ought not to be there.

Cough is a symptom belonging to a variety of complaints; it attends a slight inflammation of the mucous
membrane, or the throat and air passages, as when
we have a cold as we say. It attends also inflammations of the lungs, bronchitis, chronic and acute, pleurisy, and diseases of the heart; it may also be merely
spasmodic or nervous, as happens not unfrequently in
hysteria; but it is a symptom belonging more especially to pulmonary consumption. It is to be regarded,
as before remarked, as a healthful symptom; or, in other
words, it is a normal effort of nature, when it is not
purely nervous, to expel some offending substance
from the throat and lungs; although some old and
feeble persons laboring under chronic bronchitis, with
profuse secretions from the mucous membrane, have
not strength to cough the phlegm up, and so die, suffo-
cated in the effort.

Hooping-cough is not easily mistaken by those who have ever heard it.

Spasmodic cough occurs in adults. It comes by turns, and is violent, "tearing persons in pieces," like hooping-cough. It often arises evidently from sympathy with derangement of the stomach and digestive organs. It may, perhaps, also be united with a certain degree of inflammation of the air passages, but if so, it is not at all proportionate to the latter, being much greater than what ordinarily occurs.

The *Nervous* or *hysterical cough* is a verys ingular affection, and has often misled patients and their friends, and even the medical attendant, to think that it was a matter indicative of positive consumption. It happens oftenest in cases of young women who have not good general health. We see such persons coughing day after day, month after month, and year after year, and yet they grow no worse. They complain that every time they take in air they cough. It is loud, harsh, dry, more like a bark than a cough; sometimes it is more incessant; at other times it occurs in paroxysms which is doubtless often more annoying to hear than to suffer. I need hardly add, that in order to cure this cough we have only to remedy the affection which gives rise to it; and it should be particularly remembered, although often a comparatively trifling affair in the beginning, it is liable to end in affections of the throat and wind-pipe, and not unfrequently brings on consumption, and so destroys the patient.

The short, dry, hacking cough occurs often in the incipient stages of consumption. It may also be caused by an elongated palate, by irritation of the fauces and throat, by febrile affection, and sometimes in persons who appear to be in no appreciable way diseased.

The *aphonic cough*, signifying that which is feeble or whispering, depends on the same causes which produce aphonia, or loss of voice. In the vocal functions, it occurs in severe and extensive ulcerations of the throat, and in extreme debility arising from whatever cause.

A *stridulous, barking, wheezing*, or *whistling cough* is such as occurs in that very dangerous affection, the croup. It occurs also sometimes at the beginning of catarrh and measles. It is seldom witnessed in patients above twelve or thirteen years of age.

A *loose cough* is such as occurs in the advanced stages of colds. In consumption, in the latter stages of lung-fever, and sometimes in old age, it is caused, as its name expresses. by the presence of a loose fluid, such as mucous, purulent mucous, or pus. In colds, it is a favorable symptom.

The *hoarse, loud, dry, forcible cough* is such as exists in the early stages of pulmonary colds, and does not appear to be caused by the presence of foreign matter in the throat or lungs.

The *asthmatic cough* is that which occurs in asthma, and is to be considered as of the spasmodic kind.

The *amphoric*, or *hollow cough* has a deep reverberating sound, and is caused by large quantities of fluid matter coming from extensive cavities in the substance of the lungs. It is a striking symptom of the more advanced stages of pulmonary consumption.

Pregnancy is sometimes attended with cough, which may come in severe paroxysms, or, in other words, a spasmodic cough.   In other cases, it may be almost constant, and what is called short and teasing.   This cough may be dry, or a tough viscid fluid may be expectorated.   If it is not cured by attention to the general health, it is extremely apt to bring on abortion.   This cough, although it generally ceases suddenly after delivery, may be brought back again by carelessness, and the taking of cold.   In such cases, if a predisposition to consumption exists, the disease may then be very easily excited.

Cough is generally, though not always, one of the earliest indications of pulmonary consumption, and is consequently the first symptom which excites the attention of the patient and his relatives.   During the first weeks or months, and in some cases years, it may be slight, occurring mainly in the morning.   It appears often to arise simply from irritation in the region of the throat, hence it does not excite alarm.   I would by no means frighten people at every little symptom of cough they may experience.   I would not have them become nervous, and imagine that because they have a cough they must necessarily pass into consumption; but at the same time, I would have every one remember that *coughing is never a symptom of health.*   A person who coughs is not entirely well; and consequently no pains should be spared to arrest, if possible, this symptom; and here I am constrained to remark that in no one thing is it more important to begin in season.   As Poor Richard says, " a stitch in time saves nine," and if this principle is an important one in the common affairs of life, how much more so in matters of health !

When this early cough has continued for a time, longer or shorter, according to the case, the individual finds that after any particular exertion, such as running up stairs, speaking, reading, singing, or laughing for some time, he becomes more troubled with the cough, and the expectoration increases. As a general rule, these symptoms increase exactly in the same proportion as the disease. Cases, however, may occur in which the cough is very slight through the whole period of consumption, and in a few rare cases it has been known to appear only a few days before death. Even where tuberculous excavations of the lungs exist to a considerable extent, the cough may often be absent altogether in the disease. "It is not sufficiently known," says Portal, "that consumption may exist without the slightest cough. The lungs of consumptive patients have often been destroyed by suppuration (the formation of pus), without their having experienced the least degree of cough." Various writers have mentioned cases of this kind.

Dyspnœa, or difficulty of breathing.—This may arise from a variety of causes, such as feebleness of the heart, nervous debility, and a deranged state of the general health. It is not to be much relied on as an indication of consumption. Dyspnœa is, however, more frequently present in this disease than is generally believed. There is almost always more or less of it in consumption; but it occurs also in a variety of other complaints. On the whole, this symptom always demands attention. It is unattended with pain, is slow and gradual in its increase, and so may be little noticed for a considerable time at first. Asthma, which is necessarily attended with dyspnœa, is supposed often to cure consumption, or, in other words, if a person is attacked with the former disease he does not sink with the latter.

Expectoration.—Both patients and physicians have been in the habit of looking a good deal to the matter thrown off from the lungs in pulmonary disease. The matter expectorated, however, is not so sure a guide as has been often supposed. The quantity of matter thrown off is by no means so sure an indication of the real degree to which the disease has manifested itself in any particular case. It may be very small, while at the same time the lungs are crowded with tubercles, many of which are already in a state of ulceration. It may, on the other hand, be quite extensive, often large, when in fact the disease has made but little progress. Formerly it was imagined—and the opinion is yet prevalent, to a considerable extent, even among practitioners of medicine—that if real pus, or purulent matter, such as sinks in water, be thrown off, the case must necessarily be one of tuberculous consumption ; but it is now well known that such is not the fact. Genuine pus is often secreted from the mucous membrane of the air passages at the end of an attack of simple bronchitis, and also of a common cold. Still, I regard that the throwing off of heavy purulent matter, and such as has an offensive odor, is generally to be looked upon as an unfavorable symptom. It denotes, evidently, a depraved state of the general health. Whether the test be one of consumption or otherwise, it is a better symptom for the matter expectorated to float upon the top of water rather than sink.

It is often a matter of interest, both to the patient and the physician, to be able to ascertain whether pus does actually exist in a given case. Dr. Cullen has given the following excellent rules in his "First Lines of the Practice of Physic," Dublin edition, 1784, vol. ii. p. 224:

" 1. From the color of the matter ; as mucous is naturally transparent, and pus always opaque. When mucous becomes opaque, as it sometimes does, it becomes white, yellow, or greenish ; but the last-mentioned color is hardly ever so remarkable in mucous as in pus.

" 2. From the consistence ; as mucous is more viscid and coherent, and pus less so, and may be said to be more friable. When mucous is thrown into water, it is not readily diffused, but remains united in uniform and circular masses ; but pus, in the same circumstances, though not readily diffused, does not remain uniformly united, and by a little agitation is broken into ragged fragments.

" 3. From the odor ; which is seldom perceived in mucous, but frequently in pus. It has been proposed to try the odor of the matter expectorated by throwing it upon live coals ; but in such a trial, both mucous and pus give out a disagreeable smell, and it is not easy to distinguish between them.

" 4. From the specific gravity compared with water ; and, indeed, it is usual for the mucous of the lungs to swim on the surface of water, and for pus to sink in it. But in this we may sometimes be deceived, as pus which has entangled a great deal of air may swim, and mucous that is free from air may sink.

5

" 5. From the mixture which is discernible in the matter brought up ; for if a yellow or greenish matter appears, surrounded with a quantity of transparent or less opaque and less colored matter, the more strongly colored matter may be generally considered as pus ; as it is not easy to understand how one portion of the mucous of the lungs can be very considerably changed while the rest of it is very little so, or remains in its ordinary state.

" 6. From the admixture of certain substances with the matter thrown out from the lungs.   To this purpose we are informed, by the experiments of the late Mr. Charles Darwin : " That the vitriolic acid dissolves both mucous and pus, but 'more readily the former ; that, if water be added to such a solution of mucous, this is separated, and either swims on the surface, or, divided into flocculi, is suspended in the liquor ; whereas, when water is added to a like solution of pus, this falls to the bottom, or by agitation is diffused so as to exhibit a uniformly turbid liquor ; that a solution of the caustic fixed alkali, after some time, dissolves mucous, and generally pus ; and if water be added to such solutions the pus is precipitated, but the mucous is not.   From such experiments it is supposed that pus and mucous may be certainly distinguished from each other.

" 7. From the expectorations being attended with a hectic fever.   A catarrh, or expectoration of mucous, is often attended with fever, but never, so far as I have observed, with such a fever as I am presently to describe as a hectic.   This, in my opinion, is the most certain mark of a purulent state in some part of the body; and if others have thought differently, I am persuaded that it has been owing to this, that, presuming upon the mortal nature of a confirmed or purulent pthisis, they have considered every case in which a recovery has happened as a catarrh only; but that they may have been mistaken in this, I have shown elsewhere."

Dr. Marshall Hall has given very clear and concise explanations of the different characters of expectoration, as witnessed in different diseases, and which are the following:

"In a state of health, the natural saliva and mucous are transparent and colorless, and they generally remain so in the incipient stages of pulmonary diseases.

"When the sputa consists of mucous, which is thick, whitish, and opaque, during common pulmonary catarrh, it indicates a subsidence of the inflammation. It is sometimes yellowish or greenish, when the disease is prolonged.

"When the spittle is of a rusty red color, viscid, heaped in small masses, and adherent to the vessel into which it is discharged, the disease is pneumonia. It is also sometimes brown or yellowish in this disease.

"When liquid blood, of a fresh, florid, and frothy appearance, is thrown off by an expiratory effort in any considerable quantity, the case is one of hæmoptysis. It shows, in most cases, the existence of tubercles in the lungs, but may take place under the influence of other causes, such as catamenial irregularities, aneurism of the aorta, and external accidents. Pulmonary hæmorrhage, when slight, probably proceeds from exhalation from the mucous membrane; when more serious, from the vesicular texture, and in rare cases from the rupture or division of a blood-vessel.

"When pus is expectorated, the disease may be bronchitis, pneumonia, or phthisis. The characteristic sputum, often seen in advanced phthisis, has received the French name *pelatanne*, which has been rendered in English by the word *nummulated*. It appears in roundish masses, with shred-like edges, floating in a clear, transparent liquid. The taste is often sweetish, and the smell nauseous. But it is in some cases extremely difficult to distinguish the pus of phthisis from that of chronic catarrh.

"When chalky or calcareous concretions are coughed up, they mostly indicate tubercules or phthisis, usually in a more chronic form. Tuberculous matter is sometimes coughed up in the same disease. When the spittle is extremely fœtid, and accompanied with a putrid odor of the breath, the disease is gangrene of the lungs.

"The expectoration of young children cannot be examined, from the circumstance that the substances raised are immediately swallowed by them.

"The act of expectoration fails to take place when there is a want of sufficient sensibility in the mucous membrane, or the diseased part, to excite coughing. This happens in the lethargic and the moribund, giving rise to the well-known rattling sound in the throat, so often heard in these cases. For the same reason expectoration is suspended during sleep, and takes place in increased quantity on waking. Some patients voluntarily avoid expectoration as long as possible, on account of pain or fatigue attending the exertion of coughing."

CHAPTER XII.

Symptoms of consumption continued.—Perspiration.—This occurs
more particularly in the advanced stages of the disease.—Hectic
fever.—Thirst.—This is not always present in consumption.—The
pulse.—It is always accelerated in this disease.—Diarrhœa.—Emaciation.—Swelling of the limbs.—Aphthæ, or sore mouth.—Pains
in the chest.—The nails.—The hair.—Nervousness.—The intellect.—Delirium.—Cessation of menstruation.—Pregnancy as affecting consumption.—Practical deductions to be drawn from the foregoing description of the symptoms of consumption.

Perspiration.—Perspiration, or sweating, is a prominent symptom of consumption in its latter stages;
and is one of so much importance, that it deserves
special consideration. It occurs generally, though
not in all cases. According to Louis, it occurs in
nine tenths of those who die of phthisis.

Perspiration in consumption occurs chiefly in the
night-time; but in the more advanced stages of the
disease, it may occur whenever the patient sleeps. It
comes on most toward morning. Especially if the
patient takes a late or second sleep, remaining in the
same bed, he will be liable to suffer from profuse
sweating.

Although perspiration occurs generally in the advanced stages of pulmonary consumption, it is occasionally seen in its more early periods. But it is then
much less in quantity, and is often so little that the
patient scarcely takes any notice of it.

Perspiration, hectic fever, frequent pulse, and emaciations are sometimes the only symptoms of pulmonary disease. Whenever we meet with tl ese symptoms in a scrofulous or tuberculous constitution, it will be well for us to examine carefully as to whether pulmonary consumption does not already exist. Any state of the system in which there is great debility, may be attended with copious night sweats, and this when tuberculous consumption does not exist. Thus, in the earlier periods of nursing, a mother of delicate constitution may experience sweats. We see the same in many fevers, and in a variety of diseases; but in general there will be no great difficulty in ascertaining whether the perspiration be caused by real consumption. If arising from other causes, it is not so persistent; it sooner leaves the patient. I shall explain elsewhere the method of mitigating, and in most cases curing the night sweats, which are so troublesome and debilitating in pulmonary consumption.

Hectic fever.—This we may consider as the cause of the symptom which I have just been considering, namely, perspiration. It comes on slowly and insidiously at first, and is often, for a considerable time, so slight as not to elicit the patient's attention. A practiced observer will, however, have no difficulty in detecting it. It may be ascertained by the pulse, even in its earliest stages, as well as by some slight augmentation of the color of the cheeks. The respiration also becomes somewhat more hurried and difficult. It varies much in degree, in different stages of tne disease, in the same individual, and also in different cases. Some have very little of it, while others are

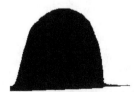

very much troubled with i . It is perhaps liable to more variation than any other prominent symptom in this disease As in all other attacks of feverishness, the patient often experiences sensations of chilliness. These are more common in the evenings. As the disease progresses, the intensity of these sensations increases, and amounts, in some cases, to almost an ague. This is succeeded by heat of the skin during the night; especially is it attended with ncrease of heat and dryness in the feet and hands. Sometimes, too, there will be an exacerbation of the hectic in the earlier part of the day, as toward noon. After a time, longer or shorter, according to the case, the paroxysms of febrile excitement become stronger, and the heat more generally diffused over the surface.

Thirst.—This symptom is usually experienced to a greater or less extent in consumption. Feverishness in this, as in all other diseases, must necessarily, I suppose, cause more or less thirst. The fever of consumption does not, as a general fact, rise at any time to a very great extent, it being chronic in its character; and hence thirst does not exist in a very great degree. I think thirst will seldom be found wholly absent, in cases of consumption. Dr. Clark has seldom seen it so, although Louis tells us he found it wanting in one fourth of his cases.

Pulse.—When we are called to examine a case in which consumption is suspected, if we find the pulse considerably more frequent than natural, and that there are no other reasons by which to account for this phenomenon, we have reason to believe that pulmonary mischief has already commenced its insidious work. On the other hand, if we find the pulse habitually at a normal standard--that is, from sixty to eighty pulsations in a minute, which includes the average of that of adults—we are to consider it as a favorable omen; still there are persons of tuberculous consumption, who have habitually a slow, languid circulation, and which in some cases continues so until the patient is perhaps far gone in the disease; but these cases are only exceptions to the general rule. In estimating the pulse in any given case, it is desirable, if possible, to know what has been the frequency or number of beats per minute when the individual was in health. The pulse varies considerably in different persons. While that of one may range from sixty to sixty-five a minute, that of another may average from seventy to seventy-five, or even eighty; consequently, what might be natural in one case, and no increase upon the healthy standard, would be a decided augmentation in another. It will be found, I think, that persons of a scrofulous and tuberculous tendency have, as a rule, a more rapid circulation, and consequently a quicker habit of pulse than those who are not so disposed.

Diarrhœa.—This symptom does not generally occur as a distinct mark of consumption until the disease is far advanced; in some cases it occurs a few days only before death, and sometimes, though rarely, it is entirely wanting. In one eighth of Louis' cases, he found diarrhœa commenced with the disease and continued till death; in the majority, it occurred in the latter stages; in others, during the last days of life only; and in four among 112 cases it never appeared.

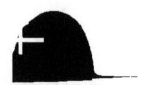

Diarrhœa is to be considered one of the most important of the symptoms of consumption; and which often, if not generally, exercises as great an influence over its progress as the expectoration does. The wasting of the flesh, the debility, and the rapidity of the disease, are generally proportionate to the severity of the diarrhœa.

This symptom often proves one of the most distressing with which the poor patient is afflicted in this disease. It is attended frequently with severe pains before, and a deadly sensation of sinking immediately after, each evacuation.

The cough and expectoration appear sometimes to be diminished by the frequency and quantity of these discharges. And pains of the chest are likewise sometimes rendered less; but, on the other hand, the extreme debility, the extreme sensation of sinking and exhaustion which are experienced, more than counterbalance.

It is a remarkable fact in consumption, that in persons who have been long subject to constipation, the bowels become exceedingly regular, and apparently healthy in their action, after consumption has become to a certain degree developed.

" The fact that the wasting and loss of strength in consumption correspond with the number and frequency of evacuations," Dr. Clark observes, "suggests a wholesome and not unnecessary caution concerning the employment of active purgatives, even in the early stages of consumption, and of mild aperients in large doses as the disease advances, since they reduce the strength, and may bring on diarrhœa before it would

5*

otherwise have occurred. I have seen," continues this writer, " a tablespoonful of castor-oil throw a consumptive patient into an alarming state of debility."

As a symptom indicative of consumption, diarrhœa is of no importance, inasmuch as it does not occur until after the disease has made considerable progress.

Emaciation.—This is to be considered as an important symptom of this disease. If there is no evident cause for it other than tuberculous disease, and if it is accompanied .by rapid pulse, loss of strength, and frequency of breathing, there is always reason to believe that tuberculous disease of the lungs already exists.

.In some cases, the derangement of the digestive organs, which is always present to a greater or less extent in consumption, is often regarded as the principal cause of the wasting of flesh ; in these cases, let persons do what they will to maintain the digestive organs in a healthy condition, and eat as freely and liberally as they may of the best and most nourishing food, the wasting yet goes on, and in spite of all that can be done. In persons about the middle period of life, as from forty to fifty, Dr. Clark regards emaciation as one of the earliest symptoms of consumption, even where there was no frequency of pulse, no cough, no marked dyspnœa, nor any other symptom to draw attention to the state of the lungs.

Emaciation, it will be understood, may occur from a variety of causes, so that it would be unwise for every person who may become debilitated and lose flesh to imagine at once that he has necessarily consumption. Still, where there is an hereditary predispo-

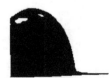

sition to this disease, a manifest wasting of the flesh should always be looked upon with suspicion.

Swelling of the limbs.—This symptom may be caused by any thing which materially debilitates the system. When it happens in a curable disease, as it sometimes does, as after an attack of fever, cholera, dysentery, etc., it is curable, provided the original malady be so; but when it happens in consumption, it is in general to be considered as a sure prognostic that the disease is approaching to its fatal termination. It is supposed to be an invariable attendant in the last stages of this disease.

Aphthæ, or sore mouth.—Generally a week or two before death, and as one of the last in the long catalogue of maladies which afflict the consumptive patient, the mouth becomes sore. Small, roundish, pearl-color vesicles appear upon the lips, within the mouth and throat, and extend probably into the intestinal canal. These are apt to slough or throw off matter to a greater or less extent as death approaches. Sometimes this symptom is productive of little inconvenience, but oftener it causes great irritation and tenderness of the mouth and throat, and proves a source of no inconsiderable suffering. We cannot, of course, expect much from remedial means in this complaint.

Pain in the chest.—Pains are not unfrequently experienced in the thoracic cavity. In pleurisy, chronic and acute, we have them, especially severe in the latter; so in rheumatism of the chest, in a common cold, too, where there is no danger whatever of tuberculous consumption, persons experience pain or coughing. Acute pain rarely attends the early stages of pulmonary phthisis; as the disease advances, it becomes generally a more prominent symptom, and some suffer a good deal with it. It is most severe on the side most affected. Pain experienced in the upper part of the chest and shoulders is sometimes indicative of the coming on of pulmonary disease, although the symptom may be so slight as not to elicit any particular attention to the patient. Indeed, often he will not mention it at all unless his attention were called to it. Such a pain may easily be confounded with rheumatism. Indeed, this early pain appears more like that of rheumatism than any thing else; and in many cases the most experienced observers will not be able to determine positively to which class it belongs. In either case, however, the indications of treatment would be the same, that is to fortify and invigorate the general health.

The nails.—In the latter stages of consumption we observe—oftenest in the cases of females, I think—an incurvated state of the nails. There is, at the same time, a rounded appearance of the last joint of the fingers. The ends of the fingers also appear to be larger than is natural.

The hair.—Owing to general debility, the wasting of the constitution, and consequent impoverishing of the skin, on the health of which the good condition of the hair so much depends, this latter not unfrequently falls off in the later stages of pulmonary disease.

Nervousness.—The patient not unfrequently becomes nervous, peevish, and irritable, even in the early stages of the malady. As the disease advances, irritability of temper and feelings, and timidity, increases.

The intellect.—It is a singular circumstance that the mind usually remains clear until the very last of this fearful disease. We find, too, that patients are ever ready *to catch at straws;* and we can seldom convince them of their danger. Where we have reason to suspect consumption, I regard it as one of the worst possible signs if the patient has no fear whatever of the disease. He thinks that he has only a little cold, which he will soon be able to throw off. He converses about his business, and prospects in life, as if he were absolutely certain of getting well; and this delusion goes on, in many cases, until the very last. On the other hand, if we find a feeble person who is continually imagining that he has the disease, and that he is certain soon to die of it, we have reason to suspect that he has only hypochondria, arising from a bad state of the general health.

Delirium.—If the feverishness runs high, or is not properly managed by remedial means, delirium sometimes comes on near the last.

Cessation of menstruation.—Cessation of this function in females is one of the common accompaniments of consumption. Let it be remembered, however, that suppression of the menses may arise from a variety of causes other than pulmonary disease. Those females who are undergoing a vigorous course of water-treatment, not unfrequently experience cessation of this function for months, and even a whole year or more, and at the same time are steadily improving in their general health. So, too, pregnancy may arrest menstruation, or the simply taking of a cold. But if a person has had for a length of time cough, the raising of purulent matter from the lungs, sweating at night, and the other accompaniments of consumption, and then with all these, if menstruation ceases, it is to be regarded a most unfavorable omen.

Pregnancy as affecting consumption.—It is an unfortunate thing for a consumptive mother to bring forth young; and it is a remarkable fact that females inclined to consumption are apt to be very prolific. Not unfrequently pregnancy occurs even in the advanced stages of pulmonary disease. It is apparently arrested in its course for the time. Possibly, in some cases, pregnancy, with its concomitant circumstances, may effect either a partial or a total cure of the disease; but I think it must far oftener happen that it only hastens on to a more rapid and fearful termination the awful disease.

Some of the more important of the practical deductions to be drawn from the foregoing description of the symptoms of pulmonary consumption are the following:

1. That pulmonary hæmorrhage, although sometimes a fatal symptom, is in general not so alarming an occurrence as is generally supposed; but that it always indicates a wrong state of things in the general health, and, as a consequence, demands special care and attention.

2. That bronchitis, or inflammation, whether acute or chronic, of the mucous membranes of the bronchial tubes, and also common sore throat, are frequent forerunners of a tuberculous disease.

3. That a cough is not necessarily an alarming symptom, but is one, however, which should always be regarded with suspicion, especially by those who are born of consumptive parents, or in whom there is a strong predisposition to pulmonary disease.

4. That we are not to regard purulent matter as being indicative necessarily of incurable disease; yet the expectoration of such matter is always to be looked upon as being a more unfavorable symptom than if mucous and light frothy expectoration be thrown off.

5. That dyspnœa, or difficult breathing, although a frequent symptom of pulmonary consumption, is also frequently to be observed in other maladies.

6. That pure asthma and pulmonary consumption do not, as a rule, go together; that an attack of the latter appears sometimes to cure the former.

7. That night sweats, although they occur in any condition of the system, attended with great debility, are always to be looked upon with caution, in regard to pulmonary disease.

8. That hectic fever, although slight in some cases, is one of the most common symptoms of this disease.

9. That thirst is not usually a prominent symptom.

10. That diarrhœa, emaciation, swelling of the limbs, and extreme soreness of the mouth and throat are to be looked upon as very unfavorable omens.

11. That pains in the chest, appearing at first to be only slight, and of a rheumatic nature, but afterward increasing in severity as the disease advances, generally attend this disease.

12. That extreme debility is one of its most prominent symptoms.

13. That the individual generally becomes very nervous, feverish, and irritable

14. That the intellect usually remains clear.

15. That delirium comes on a little before death in some cases, especially if the fever be not properly treated.

16. That suppression of the menstrual function is a frequent symptom of females toward the fatal close of the disease.

17. That the cessation of the menses may also attend a variety of circumstances where no pulmonary disease is present.

18. That pregnancy and nursing appear, in general, to check consumption for the time, and in some cases to cure it altogether ; but that, as a general fact, these circumstances tend only to hasten the final termination of the disease.

CHAPTER XIII.

Causes of consumption.—The predisposing and the exciting causes of disease.—Hereditary predisposition.—Transmission of physiological and pathological qualities from parent to child.—Consumption not always hereditary.—Ways in which it may be brought on in the system.—Intermarriage as affecting pulmonary consumption. —Relations should not intermarry.—Reasons why.—Is consumption a contagious disease ?—Authorities quoted.—Relation of scrofula to consumption.—Important and instructive facts concerning the causes and the prevention of consumption.

THE causes of consumption, as of most other diseases, are of two classes, the *predisposing* and the *exciting*.

Predisposing causes are such as tend to bring about a certain state of things in the system, in which it is more liable, under certain circumstances, to take on a particular form of disease.

Exciting causes are such as occasion a development of any certain disease to which the system has already been predisposed. Thus, a person of consumptive habits may be exposed to severe wet and cold, by which consumption is brought on. Wet and cold are here the exciting causes. If several persons were subjected to a long and severe exposure to cold, one might experience, as a consequence, inflammation of the lungs ; another, pleurisy ; another, inflammation of the bowels ; another, gout ; another, rheumatism ; another, erysipelas ; another, a general fever ; and still another might escape unharmed. The character of the disease, in each of these cases, would be in ac-

cordance with the predisposition existing in each individual case.

Hereditary predisposition.—It is a familiar fact to
all, that children always inherit, to a greater or less
degree, the looks, conformation, and general constitution of their parents. It will be found, I think, a general rule, that daughters resemble the male parent
most, both in appearance and general constitution,
and sons the female parent. If this be true—and I
think facts of observation warrant me in asserting it—
a daughter has more to fear from consumption if the
disease existed on the father's side, than if on the
mother's ; and the son the contrary. But if the disease be farther back, as among the grandparents, the
daughter has more to fear if the disease have been on
the grandmother's side, and the contrary of the son.

I know of no author who has put forth these views,
but I think, notwithstanding, that they will be found
to be in accordance with the facts.

Professor Sweetser, in his work on consumption
(page 96), gives a striking instance in proof of the
transmission of certain qualities from parent to child.
He observes :

"An interesting fact was related to me, a few years
since, by Professor Zerah Colburn, the gentleman who
was so extensively known, in early life, for his extraordinary powers of calculation. One of his parents
(his father) had a supernumerary finger and toe on
each hand and foot, which malformation he inherited,
being born with six fingers on his upper, and six toes
on his lower extremities. Some of his brothers dis-
played the same peculiarity, others not. The extra

fingers were cut off in infancy. The lady whom he married was a distant connection of his own, and inherited exactly the same malformation. She had born him three children, two of whom were twins, and all with a supernumerary finger and toe on each hand and on each foot. Desirous of learning some more particulars in regard to this peculiarity, and especially whether it would continue to be transmitted to his offspring, I recently addressed a communication on the subject to Professor Colburn, to which he kindly replied, acquainting me with the following additional and interesting facts, which I will give in his own language: ' I do not know at what period this peculiarity was imported into this country. It came, I believe, from Scotland, in the name of Kendall. From the Kendalls it came into the family of Green, by marriage. My grandfather married a Green, and thus it got into our family. How many, if any, of my uncles had this mark, I know not. My father had it on each hand and foot; of his children, one brother and myself have it complete. One other brother has *one* odd finger; he has two children, twins, and both completely furnished with odd fingers and toes. The other brothers and sisters have it not, either themselves or in their children. My wife is great-granddaughter of my grandfather; her mother has one finger and one toe extra. This fact accounts for her being born with the full complement of supernumerary fingers and toes; they were cut off at her birth, by the attending physician. Since I saw you I have been favored with another daughter, with like accoutrements, and have not any doubt but, even though I had as many as Gideon of old, by my present wife, they would all show alike in this respect, and be, like my four daughters now, six fingered and six toed. The descendants of Kendall generally have this distinction, or can tell of some kinsman who has.' "

The world is full of examples showing the effects which peculiar qualities or predispositions of parents may entail upon their offspring.

Consumption not always hereditary.—It is to be observed that consumption, although often an hereditary disease, is not always so. The new-born child is sometimes affected with tubercles, even where no taint of the sort can be traced in the family. Laennec observed that "numerous families are at times destroyed by the disease, whose parents were never affected by it." Cases have been known in which the parents have both died at a very advanced age, but previously having buried a large family of children, all of whom died of consumption. Laennec has mentioned an instance in which the father and mother died upward of eighty years of age, and of acute maladies, after having seen fourteen children, born healthy, and without any indications of a predisposition to consumption, successively carried off by it, between the ages of fifteen and thirty-five.

Dr. Clark also informs us, that instances have come under his observation, " where whole families have fallen victims to tuberculous consumption, while the parents themselves enjoyed good health, to an advanced age, and were unable to trace the existence of the disease in their families, for generations back."

How are we to account for facts like these ?—Con-

sumption had a beginning somewhere. This origi-
nated, doubtless, in consequence of man's physical
transgression. We cannot believe that the wise and
benevolent Creator would bring upon man so dreadful
a disease, through causes which are not, as a general
principle, under his control. True, a child may inherit the disease from its parents, and so be unable to
ward it off; still, its parents or its parents' parents
were accountable for the disease ; so that we have, in
this matter of hereditary predisposition, an illustration
of the principle that "the iniquities of the fathers are
visited upon their children unto the third and fourth
generation." Should we observe carefully, I have
no doubt we might trace, in our great and unhealthy
cities, many cases of consumption, where the more
healthy parents, who were born and reared up in the
more healthy country, had no tendency whatever to
the disease. A multitude of causes may operate, a
considerable time, upon both parents, which will bring
on the disease, where no predisposition to it has existed.

A depraved state of the general health in the
mother, before and during pregnancy, does often un-
questionably exercise a very deleterious influence upon the new being whose life is so intimately connected
with her own; and by this means, we have every
reason to believe, tubercles are sometimes formed.

There is an important consideration—one which
should be deeply pondered, and for which we should
be ever thankful to the Author of our being, that inasmuch as man, by his physical wrong-doing, brings
upon himself so terrible a malady as consumption, so

may he, by a correct course of physical management, ward off the disease ; in other words, as the tendency of nature is ever downward, under bad influences, so, on the other hand, is her tendency ever upward, under the operation of good influences.

Intermarriage as affecting consumption.—"Members of families," says Dr. Clark, "already predisposed to tuberculous disease, should at least endeavor to avoid matrimonial alliance with others in the same condition ; but above all they should avoid the too common practice of intermarrying with their own immediate relatives—a practice at once a fertile source of scrofula, and a sure mode of deteriorating the intellectual and physical powers, and eventually the means of extinguishing a degenerated race."

It has always been found injurious among the inferior animals to allow those which are in any way diseased to breed in-and-in, as the term is. So well apprised of this fact are breeders of animals, that they are in the habit of introducing frequent *crosses* among their flocks. If man is so careful in rearing his horses, oxen, sheep, and swine, how much more so should he be in the propagation of his own species.

The remark, that it is a sign of bad luck to marry a relative, has long since grown into a proverb, and, as is true with most other popular proverbs, it is based in wisdom drawn from observation. It was long since observed that, in unions between blood-relations, the various imperfections existing in families, and their morbid predispositions, are exceedingly liable to be perpetuated ; and in consequence of the impulse received from both of the parents, are greatly aggra-

vated in the offspring. The degeneracy of many royal families might be cited in proof of this doctrine.

Burton says, " I think it has been ordered by God's special providence, that, in all ages, there should be, once in six hundred years, a transmigration of nations, to amend and purify their blood, as we alter seed upon our land;" and Sir Humphrey Davy remarks. " You saw, in the decline of the Roman empire, a people enfeebled by luxury, worn out by excess, overrun by rude warriors; you saw the giants of the North and East mixing with the pigmies of the South and West. An empire was destroyed, but the seeds of moral and physical improvement in the new race were sown; the new population, resulting from the alliances of the men of the North with the women of the South, was more vigorous, more full of physical power, and more capable of intellectual exertion than their apparently ill-suited progenitors; and the moral effects are final causes of the migration of races, the plans of conquest and ambition which have led to revolutions and changes of kingdoms, designed by man for such different objects, have been the same in their ultimate results—that of improving by mixture the different families of men. An Alaric, or an Attila, who marched with legions of barbarians for some gross view of plunder or ambition, is an instrument of divine power to effect a purpose of which he is wholly unconscious— he is carrying a strong race to improve a weak one, and giving energy to a debilitated population; and the deserts he makes in his passage will become, in another age, cultivated fields; and the solitude he produces will be succeeded by a powerful and healthy

population.   The results of these events, in the moral
and political world, may be compared to those produced in the vegetable kingdom by the storms and
heavy gales so usual at the vernal equinox, the time
of the formation of the seed ; the pollen or farina of
one flower is thrown upon the pistil of another, and
the crossing of varieties of plants, so essential to the
vegetable world, produced."

If persons of consumptive tendency marry at all,
the opposite party should by all means be as free as
possible from all predisposition to this complaint ; and
the healthier and more hardy in other respects the
better.   That the Mosaic law relating to marriage of
relatives was founded in wisdom, facts abundantly
prove.

Is consumption a contagious disease?—It may be,
and probably is true, that all severe and dangerous
diseases have a tendency, greater or less, to produce
their kind.   It is well known that hysteria, epilepsy,
St. Vitus' dance, and catalepsy may be communica-
ted by sympathy.   The same also might, probably
with truth, be said of cholera, and various other diseases.   But that consumption is contagious, or that it
is transmitted directly from one person to another, in
any proper acceptation of the term contagious, cannot,
I think, be proved.   If we take into consideration the
great frequency of consumption and other pulmonary
complaints confounded with it, we need not be at a
loss to account for the seeming transmission of it from
one individual to another, if one fourth, one fifth, or
even one sixth part of the population die of consump
tion.

Many cases will necessarily occur, however, where one individual will seem to take it from another. But we see husbands nurse their wives, and wives their husbands, parents their children, and children their parents, and yet the survivors do not seem to fall into consumption immediately afterward, unless there has been beforehand a strong predisposition to it. If the husband or his wife dies of this disease, it will, I think, very seldom be found that the other party falls a victim to the disease, unless it has existed beforehand in the system.

In Languedoc, Spain, and Portugal consumption is believed to be contagious, and, in accordance with this idea, the clothes of patients who have died of the disease are there burned by the civil authorities. "Morgagni was so frightened at the contagiousness of this disease," says Dr. Elliotson, "that he never opened the body of a person who died of it." Dr. Morton, an English author, considers it contagious. But with very few exceptions, from the time of Hippocrates down, consumption has been considered a non-contagious disease.

Relation of scrofula to consumption.—Scrofula and consumption are reckoned by most writers as having an intimate relation. It has, indeed, been maintained that true tubercular consumption is necessarily a scrofulous disease. The term scrofula, however, is not well defined; but what is generally termed scrofula is to be regarded as being, in many cases, co-existent with, or an exciting cause of, consumption. Scrofula affects persons most who have fair hair and complexion, fine clear skin, and a predominance of

6

the sanguine temperament, such precisely as are most liable to pulmonary disease. Any thing, then, which tends to the production of scrofula, we may consider as being equally productive of tubercular consumption.

"Consumption," says Dr. Griscom, "is very often, if not always, *a symptom* of a disease which assumes different forms, and is known by the generic term SCROFULA."

Bad air as a cause of consumption and scrofula.— M. Baudelocque, a celebrated French writer, who has made the causes of scrofula a subject of careful investigation, and whose opinions have been extensively adopted by the best physicians in Europe and the United States, makes the following remarks concerning the causes of this disease:

"Invariably it will be found, on examination, that a truly scrofulous disease is caused by a vitiated air, and it is not always necessary that there should have been a prolonged stay in such an atmosphere. Often a few hours each day is sufficient, and it is thus they may live in the most healthy country, pass the greater part of the day in the open air, and yet become scrofulous, because of sleeping in a confined place, where the air has not been renewed. This is the case with many shepherds. It is usual to attribute scrofula, in their case, to exposure to storms and atmospheric changes, and to humidity. But attention has not been paid to the circumstance that they pass the night in a confined hut, which they transport from place to place, and which guarantees them against humidity; this hut has only a small door, which is closed when they enter, and remains closed also during the day ; six or eight hours passed daily in a vitiated air, and which no draught ever removes, is the true cause of their disease. I have spoken of the bad habit of sleeping with the head under the clothes, and the insalubrity of the classes where a number of children are assembled together. The repetition of these circumstances is often sufficient cause of scrofula, although they may last but for a few hours a day."

M. Baudelocque cites, in confirmation of his views, the following striking example :

" At three leagues from Amiens lies the village of Oresmeaux; it is situated in a vast plain, open on every side, and elevated more than a hundred feet above the neighboring valleys. About sixty years ago most of the houses were built of clay, and had no windows ; they were lighted by one or two panes of glass fixed in the wall ; none of the floors, sometimes many feet below the level of the street, were paved. The ceilings were low ; the greater part of the inhabitants were engaged in weaving. A few holes in the wall, and which were closed at will by means of a plank, scarcely permitted the light and air to penetrate into the workshop. Humidity was thought necessary to keep the threads fresh. Nearly all the inhabitants were seized with scrofula, and many families, continually ravaged by that malady, became extinct; their last members, as they write me, died rotten with scrofula. A fire destroyed nearly one third of the village ; the houses were rebuilt in a more salubrious manner, and by degrees scrofula became less common, and disappeared from that part. Twenty years later, another third of the village was consumed ; the same ameliora tion in building produced a like effect as to scrofula. The disease is now confined to the inhabitants of the older houses, which retain the same causes of insalubrity."

Dr. Guy, of England, in his examination before the health commissioners, affirms, that the deficient ventilation or foul air is more productive of consumption than all other causes put together. The results of his inquiries, respecting the causes of this disease, were—

" 1. Consumption is relatively more frequent in persons working in doors than those employed out of doors.

" 2. In those employments within doors, it is most frequent with men using little exertion.

" 3. It makes its attacks earlier where it is of most frequent occurrence.

" 4. It is very common in the intemperate, and in those exposed to the inhalation of dust.

" 5. It is more frequent in men than women, at least in the city of London."

According to Dr. Guy, of the three classes of men, gentlemen (including professional men), tradesmen (storekeepers), and artisans (including laborers of every class), the cases of consumption stand as the numbers 16, 28, and 30.

" From this it follows," says Dr. Griscom, " that the tradesmen of London (and they are pretty similarly circumstanced in New York, and the other cities of this country), are nearly twice as liable to consumption as the gentry. This great mortality, Dr. Guy mainly attributes to the confinement, during so many hours of every day in ill-ventilated shops. In large cities, the tradesmen and shopmen suffer occasionally from the way in which they are lodged or housed. They give

up to their business all the space they can command,
and let the upper part of their houses to lodgers, living themselves in small back rooms, connected with
their stores, which rooms are no larger or better ventilated than those of the poor. This leads to much
sickness among them. 'It is,' continues Dr. Guy,
'only within a few days that a London tradesman
gave me this account of himself: He had been originally a workman, and, having saved a little money,
opened a small store in a back street. For some years
he slept in a small, close back room, behind his shop,
and during the whole time was subject to frequent attacks of cold, with affection of the chest. These attacks were often so severe as to require medical advice
and attendance, for weeks together. He has since
moved into an open, airy situation, with ample accom-
modation for himself and family, and he is not only
rarely subject to colds, but these, when they do occur,
are readily cured by the most simple means. He
states that he saves, in this way, a large sum previously expended on medicine.' "

It is well known that farmers, who are exposed almost
constantly to the invigorating effects of air, light, and
exercise, seldom die of consumption.

"Were I to select two circumstances," says Sir
James Clark, "which influence the health, especially
during the growth of the body, more than any others,
and concerning which the public, generally at present
most ignorant of them, ought to be well informed, they
would be the proper adaptation of food to difference
of constitution, and the constant supply of pure air for
respiration '

CHAPTER XIV.

The causes of consumption continued.—Want of light.—Light as important to animal bodies as the vegetable.—Interesting and important facts in corroboration of this doctrine.—Consumption is found most among those who inhabit the darkest places of cities.—Effects of insufficiency of food.—Excessive alimentation.—Its effects illustrated by various facts.

Want of light.——As light is one of the most important agents in the growth and well-being of the vegetable productions of the earth, so, also, it is not less important in the animal. If tadpoles be nourished with proper food, and at the same time be exposed to a constantly renewed contact of water, so that their respiration may be fully carried on, while they remain in their fish-like condition, and at the same time be deprived entirely of light, their growth continues, but their metamorphosis into the condition of air-breathing animals is arrested, and they remain in the condition of a large tadpole. So the rapidity with which water-flies, and other insects of pools, undergo their transformation, is found to be much influenced by the amount of light to which they are exposed. If equal numbers of the eggs of the silkworm be preserved in a dark room, and exposed to common daylight, a much larger number of them are hatched from the latter than the former.

It has been observed, too, that a remarkable freedom from deformity is to be found among those nations that wear but little clothing, thus leaving the system more exposed to the influence of air and light; while on the other hand, those who are much confined within doors, or are born and brought up in cellars, mines, narrow and dark streets, and like places, deformity is much oftener found.

"It has been stated by Sir A. Wylie, who was long at the head of the medical staff in the Russian army," says Dr. Carpenter, "that the cures of disease, on the dark side of an extensive barrack at St. Petersburgh, have been uniformly, for many years, in the proportion of three to one, to those on the side exposed to strong light. And in one of the London hospitals, with a long range of frontage looking nearly due north and south, it has been observed that a residence in the south wards is much more conducive to the welfare of the patient, than in those on the north side of the building."

In accordance with these facts, we find that consumption goes most among the inhabitants of the dark parts of the cities. It is to be observed, too, that females, who are less exposed to light, because of their remaining more in-door than males, are also more subject to consumption. By referring to the tables of M. Benoiston de Chateauneuf, quoted in another part of this work, it will be seen that rag-pickers, stone-quarriers, stone-cutters, and carpenters, all of whom are much exposed to the influence of light, have a low average of mortality from consumption. As I have remarked elsewhere, it is well known that farmers, and all such persons as are exposed almost constantly to the open air, vigorous exercise, and light, are of all persons the most free from consumption.

Insufficiency of food.—In the old country, a want of proper food often becomes a cause of consumption. Among the poor of the European cities, where consumption is so exceedingly prevalent, meagreness of diet is to be considered as one of the most prolific among the many causes of the disease; but in our own country, an insufficient supply of food cannot properly be reckoned among the causes of consumption, although such cases may now and then happen. Even in our almshouses, which are peopled mainly by the offscouring of almost all nations, there is far more harm from excess, than from a restricted supply of nourishment.

Excess in food.—This has not generally been reckoned as among the causes of consumption; but inasmuch as excessive alimentation may become a cause of a great variety of diseases, so also, we have every reason to believe, it may become a cause of consumption. That able writer, Sir James Clark, well remarks, on this subject, that "proper food (as well as improper), when taken in excess, or of too exciting a quality, may also induce tuberculous cachexia in youth—a circumstance which is not sufficiently attended to, I may say not generally understood, even by medical men; nevertheless, I hold it to be a frequent cause of scrofula. Imperfect digestion and excitement of the digestive organs, in the one case, and inadequate supply of nourishment in the other, lead ultimately to a similar state of disease; the form and general character which it assumes may differ, but in

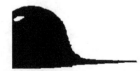

both cases the result may be the same. The adaptation of food, in quantity and quality, to the age of the individual, as well as to the powers of the digestive organs, is too little considered, and the evil consequences of this neglect are often evinced in the children of the wealthy classes, who are frequently allowed an unrestricted use of the most exciting kinds of animal food, than which there cannot be a greater error. By a too stimulating diet at this early age, the digestive organs become over-excited; the biliary and other secretions, connected with digestion, are diminished; congestion of the abdominal circulation ensues; and the skin, sympathizing with the irritation of the internal surface, becomes dry and harsh; and cutaneous eruptions, or copious perspiration, are common consequences. The ultimate effect is often tuberculous disease, which is generally attributed to imperfect nourishment; and on this erroneous view, steel and other tonics, and stimulants, are often prescribed, by which the evil is increased.

So all-pervading are the errors concerning the effects of excessive alimentation, and of too great concentration in food, in our country generally, I will proceed to remark at some length on these evils.

It is a well-ascertained law of the animal economy, that food, to be healthy, must contain a considerable portion of matter that is wholly indigestible and innutritious. Thus, Magendie, the physiologist, found that dogs, fed upon sugar, gum arabic, butter, olive-oil, and some other articles of rich or concentrated nature, each given to the animals separately, with pure water, they very soon lost their appetites, began to droop

6*

became emaciated, were attacked with ulcers, and died, invariably, within the space of four or five weeks. Fed upon superfine flour-bread and water, they lived uniformly about seven weeks, varying only a day or two. When fed upon coarse or military bread, such as contained either the whole or a considerable portion of the bran, the dogs thrived perfectly well, and were found in no respect to suffer. The same truth has often been illustrated on shipboard, at sea. In many cases, where the hay and straw have been swept overboard, it has been found that the animals, in a few days, famished, unless some innutritious substance, as the shavings of wood, was mixed with the grain given them. The animals have been observed to gnaw at the spars and timbers, or whatever wood they could lay hold of; and thus the idea was suggested, that the grain alone was of too rich a nature for their sustenance.

The same principle holds good in reference to the health of the human body; and, as a general fact, food, in civilized life, is of too concentrated a quality. This is particularly true in those parts of the world where an abundance can be had; in other words, in the more civilized and enlightened parts of the world. A host of diseases, both acute and chronic, are either caused or greatly aggravated by concentration in food. Indigestion, with its immense train of evils, constipation, loss of flesh, corpulency, nervous and general debility, torpor, and sluggishness of the general system are the principal roots of all diseases in the human family; and these are among the difficulties caused by too great richness in food. Children are often injured in this way. Mothers, in their kindness, think nothing too good for their little ones. In many parts of our country, the infant at the breast is taught to suck at its piece of pork, or other fat meat. Sugar, sugar-candy, sweetened milk, superfine bread, and rich pastries are all given for the same reason, by mothers and nurses, in their mistaken kindness. Children reared in this way can never be healthy for any considerable length of time, are generally very puny and weak, and often die within two or three years of birth. Scrofulous and other ulcers are frequently thus caused, and so also those derangements of the stomach and bowels, which so often, in spite of the best remedial means, sweep these little sufferers from their earthly existence; and this at the very time when their growing minds begin to gladden the parent's heart. There is great and prevailing error upon this subject, and happy are those parents who take it upon themselves to gain wisdom in the most important matter of food.

Sedentary and studious persons, and especially young ladies at seminaries and boarding-schools, suffer much from the effects of superfine bread, and other forms of concentrated food. Constipation, which is always attended with unpleasant results, is very common among this class of persons; one of the greatest causes of that state of health being too great richness in food.

The effects of superfine flour were strikingly illustrated in the case of a crew of seamen belonging to Providence, R. I. The narrative was quoted from Graham's Science of Human Life, and is as follows:

"Captain Benjamin Dexter, of the ship Isis, belonging to Providence, R. I., arrived from China in December, 1804. He had been about 190 days on the passage. The sea bread, which had constituted the principal article of food for his hands, was made of the best of superfine flour. He had not been long at sea before the men began to complain of languor, loss of appetite, and debility. These difficulties increased during the whole voyage, and several of the men died on the passage from debility and inanition. The ship was obliged to come to anchor about thirty miles below Providence; and such was the debility of the hands on board, that they were not able to get the ship under way again; and the owners were under the necessity of sending men down from the city of Providence to work her up. When she arrived, the owners asked Captain Dexter what was the cause of the sickness of his men, to which he answered, " The bread is too good."

Cases of similar kind have elsewhere been known to occur. Sailors, the world over, are generally furnished with brown sea bread, much to the advantage of this useful class of men, did they but know it; and their health is proverbially good while they are away from the temptations upon land. These hardy, weather-beaten men are subjected to many healthful influences other than the use of coarse bread, but, on the whole, their dietetic and other hygienic habits need greatly to be improved; still, compared with the mass of mankind, they are remarkably healthy.

Every one who is aware of the importance of a certain degree of innutritiousness in food, must lament many of the so-called improvements of modern times. Who can think of the good dishes our New England mothers used to prepare, homely and plain, as the fastidious would now consider them to be, and not desire earnestly that such days of simplicity might again return to us ? As things are, if a person travels from home, or visits among friends, almost every dish that is set before him is of a form so concentrated as to be positively injurious. At the best hotels and boarding-houses, upon the floating palaces that glide upon our waters, and in our splendid ships that traverse the seas, the evil we speak of is generally prevalent.

Now, in view of all these pernicious practices—practices, too, which are so common in our country at the present day—who does not see that the increase of that most fearful of all maladies which have ever afflicted the human race, is owing in great part to excess in quantity, and in too great richness of food. When the world has long enough quailed under the strong hand of disease, may we not hope that a better state of things will exist? that the race will **again** return to nature, and thus become free ?

CHAPTER XV.

Causes of consumption continued.—Deficient exercise.—Its effects.—
Excessive labor.—The latter a less frequent cause of disease than
the former.—Over-exertion of the lungs in public speaking, singing
and playing on wind instruments.—A due degree of exercise of the
vocal organs highly conducive to health.—Excessive mental labor.
—Erroneous notions concerning the education of the young.—
Clothing.—Females are most liable to suffer from improper dress.—
Errors of mothers on this subject.—Want of cleanliness.—Spirituous drinks.—Spirit drinkers are very liable to consumption.

Deficient exercise.—According to all well-ascertained
facts, it is found that those who are engaged in
laborious occupations, are, as a general rule, the least
liable to consumption. Farmers are proverbially free
from the disease. Sailors, also, seldom experience it.
According to the tables of M. Benoiston de Chateauneuf, drawn from observation in four of the largest
Parisian hospitals, it will be seen that those who are
engaged in the most laborious occupations, such as
blacksmiths, locksmiths, stone-sawyers, stone-cutters,
stone-quarriers, carpenters, masons, and laborers were
the most free from consumption. On the other hand,
such as were subject to in-door occupations, and
especially those in which a part of the system was
mainly exercised, such as jewelers, tailors, shoe-
makers, polishers, embroiderers, seamstresses, glove-
makers, etc., the proportion of deaths by consumption
was very large.

If a due supply of proper food and pure air is

necessary to the growth and well-being of the human body, habitual exercise in the open air is not less so. "Without exercise," says Sir James Clark, "we have abundant proof that there cannot be sound health, more particularly in early life."

Excessive labor.—This, too, may become a cause of consumption. Doubtless, among farmers of many parts of our country, the youth are in the habit of working too hard. Excessive labor, particularly at an early age, exhausts and debilitates the system, and checks the full growth and development of the body; especially when this labor is carried on in confined apartments, and in impure air, are its effects more decided. But a deficiency of physical labor, far oftener than too much, is a cause of disease.

Over-exertion of the lungs in public speaking, singing, and playing on wind instruments, etc.—A due degree of exercise of the organs of speech, the lungs, and other parts concerned in the vocal functions, is highly conducive to health. Such exercise calls the muscles of respiration into free action, thus aiding to produce a full expansion and development of the chest and lungs. But as any other part of the system may be injured by excessive exercise, so also the lungs. Violent efforts in playing on wind instruments, and in public speaking, and especially if these efforts are periodical, and at considerable intervals, are, without great care, necessarily prejudicial to those who are predisposed to pulmonary disease. But reading aloud, from day to day, and frequent public speaking, when not carried to excess, are excellent means for invigorating the lungs. It is particularly necessary here to understand how to distinguish between the use and abuse of a valuable means.

Excessive mental labor.—Too much exertion of mind, as well as of body, is not unfrequently productive of harm to the constitution. Excessive mental labor operates injuriously in two ways. First, the sensorial power of the system becomes exhausted by too long application to study and books. And secondly, the body becomes debilitated by the want of exercise in manual occupations.

The notions of many are altogether wrong, as regards education of the young. Weakly boys, parents suppose, may be sent to school and prepared for a profession. The weakly may become, too, a teacher, a clergyman, or a lawyer, or a merchant's clerk, it is supposed, while the stronger ones are kept at home upon the farm. Now this is all wrong. The professions of divinity, law, and medicine are all harder upon the constitution than the occupation of farming, or other active out-door employments. Therefore it is that the stronger should enter these professions, and not the weaker. And the professional man should remember that he can accomplish more with his brain, if he will do daily a certain amount of physical work. The elder Rev. Dr. Beecher was, we are told, in the habit daily of sawing wood for exercise ; and he holds that such exercise was indispensable, in order to success in the ministerial avocation.

Clothing.—The subject of clothing has become certainly a very common one; but yet there is, I apprehend, little danger of *overdoing* the subject. So long as people will continue to dress improperly, so long should there be those who raise their voice against the practice.

Ladies, more especially, are liable to suffer from erroneous practices in regard to clothing. Generally, too great an amount is worn; then to attend a theatre, a ball, or party, or wedding, a great change is made. Their stockings and delicate shoes are all of a sudden changed for less substantial ones. The same general change is made in the dress. Who does not know that by these improper changes cold is often taken that lasts for weeks and months, and in not a few instances becomes the foundation of incurable disease, ending, in some instances, very soon in death.

Mothers are greatly at fault in this matter. Great changes in regard to dress should never be made suddenly, even with persons in health. So impressed with the importance of this rule was one great physician, that he laid down as a maxim that all who wear flannels should, in the warmest of the summer, throw it off one day and resume it the next. Now I repeat again, there is generally far too much clothing worn; but all changes, to a less amount, should be made in connection with cool or cold bathing; and always gradual, if it may be. Many a cold is received, when, if at the making the change the cold bathing, followed by exercise, had been practiced, the individual would have been safe.

The practice of wearing dresses low at the neck is often prejudicial to health. About the waist there is worn a half a dozen or more thicknesses, while low about the neck there are none at all. At another time, perhaps, the same person will have the neck warmly clad. These changes are not good, as a general thing, and persons have often received injury by making them.

The skin is truly a breathing organ; hence clothing should never be so tight as to prevent the exposure of air to the surface. As a general fact, the more loose and flowing clothing is, the better for health.

Want of cleanliness.—Among the most filthy and degraded people of large towns and cities, we always find the most consumption and kindred diseases; hence we must set down uncleanliness as one among many of the prolific causes of consumption.

Spirituous drinks.—Spirit drinkers are often affected with a cough. This is particularly troublesome when he first rises in the morning. Any thing which injures the general health, as all forms of spirituous drinks do, and especially any thing that excites a cough, is very liable to become a cause of pulmonary disease. "While this pernicious habit," says Sir James Clark, "is one of the most powerful means of debasing the morals of the people, and of extinguishing the best feelings of human nature, it is no less fatal in destroying the physical constitution. There is good reason to believe that the abuse of spirituous liquors among the lower classes in England, is productive of consumption, and other tuberculous diseases, to an extent far beyond what is generally imagined. The bland, cadaverous aspect of the spirit drinker bespeaks the condition of his internal organs. The tale of his moral and physical degradation is indelibly written on his countenance. The evil, unfortunately, does not rest with himself by destroying his own health, but entails on his unhappy offspring the disposition to tuberculous disease."

CHAPTER XVI.

Causes of consumption continued.—Mercury.—General effects of this drug.—It exerts a very deleterious influence upon those who are predisposed to consumption.—Abuse of medicines generally as a cause of tuberculous disease.—Drugs are used to great excess by the American people.—Tea and coffee.—These injure the general health, and may therefore aid in causing tuberculous disease.— Tobacco.—Its narcotic and poisonous effects on the living body.— Hard water as a cause of disease.—Scrofula in Vermont.—Pure soft water far more healthful than that which is hard.

Mercury.—Dr. Clark observes that mercury, when used so as to affect the system, has been very generally considered as capable of inducing tuberculous disease. "I am inclined," says he, "to believe this; and therefore consider that in persons of a delicate or strumous constitution, its use requires the greatest caution and circumspection." If mercury is capable of producing dropsy, as is stated by Sir Astley Cooper, or enlargement of most of the glands of the body, as according to Dieterick, or sloughing and ulceration of the gums and throat, as according to Sir Astley Cooper and many others, or mercurial leprosy, as is stated by Moriarty, or mercurial fevers and salivation, as is stated by numerous authorities, or mercurial tremors, or palsy, as according to Dr. Christison, or mercurial wasting of the bowels, as has been often observed, or a rotting and decaying of the bones, a fact well known to medical men—I say, if mercury

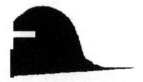

may cause all these evils, which it does, with a host of others, too numerous to mention, we may easily believe in the existence of the mercurial wasting, described by Travers as known " *by irritable circulation, extreme pallor and emaciation, and acute and rapid hectic, and an almost invariable termination in pulmonary consumption.*"

According to experiments, made in France by Couveelhier, on dogs, in which crude mercury was injected into the lungs through the air-tubes, and into the cellular textures of other organs, tubercles, with a globule of mercury in their centre, was the result.

"In the year 1810," says Dr. Sweetser, " a large quantity of quicksilver was taken from the wreck of a Spanish vessel, on board the English ship Triumph, of seventy-four guns, and the boxes principally stowed in the bread-room. Many of the bladders, in which it was confined—owing to the heat of the weather, and to having been wetted during their removal—soon rotted, and several tons of the mercury were diffused through the ship, mixing with the bread, and more or less with the other provisions. The consequence was, that very many of the officers and crew experienced severe salivations, and other deleterious effects, from the mercury that was taken into their systems, two dying from its influence ; and that nearly all the live stock, as well as cats, mice, a dog, and even a canary bird, died.

"But how did it affect the lungs? The account informs us that the mercury was very deleterious to those having any tendency to pulmonic affections ; that three men, who had previously manifested no indisposition, died of pulmonary consumption ; and that one man, who had before suffered from lung-fever, but was entirely cured, and another, who had had no pulmonic complaint before, were left behind, at Gibraltar, with confirmed phthisis."

Abuse of medicines generally.—If mercury is known to produce such disastrous results on the constitution, we may readily suppose that other powerful drugs may do the same.   Iodine, an article much used at the present day, is a substance which, when taken for a continuance, pervades the whole system, and is no doubt often a prominent cause in the development of consumption.   Those people who are the most sickly, we find, as a general fact, are most in the habit of taking medicines ; and those who take the most medicines are most liable to consumption.   If we are any where to regard the maxim of Hoffman, " avoid physic and physicians if you value health," it is in reference to tubercular consumption.

If the American people are more energetic than all other nations in money-making and general handicraft ; and if they are, on the whole, more independent than any other people, so, also, are they more persevering in the use of the thousand-and-one nostrums and quack medicines of the day.   It was well said, a few years since, by an eloquent lawyer in the legislature of the State of New York, sarcastically it is true, " that with all our keen-sightedness, adroitness, skill and ingenuity in all we undertake, we are, perhaps, the most easily humbugged nation in the world. In nothing is this alacrity to be deceived more fully manifested than in the never-ending, still-beginning, doctor-still, and still-destroying patent medicines. Perhaps one fourth of the advertising patronage of the country newspapers consists in puffing patent medicines, and this great tariff is levied on credulity afflicted with disease. If there were truth in the advertisements of a single paper, attested by the learned, the wise, and the pious, there is not a disease to which poor humanity is heir, but what is susceptible of speedy relief and ultimate cure."

Who does not know that there are, all over our States, multitudes of consumptive persons who are every day reading those infamous advertisements, which are every where put forth in this country of more newspapers than the whole world besides, and catching at the promises of the infernal quack-venders like a drowning man catching at a straw? I have just been consulted by an elderly lady of a rich family in the city of New York, who acknowledges that she has for years been watching the papers, and has tried every thing in which the advertisers have promised relief. Evidently, consumption of the lungs will soon number her days, and this, too, although she was not hereditarily predisposed to it.

Tea and coffee.—If tea and coffee are sufficient, as facts abundantly prove, to cause, in their worst forms, tremulousness, hysteria, hypochondriasis, depression of spirits, sick headache, palpitation of the heart, paleness and sallowness of complexion, and decay of the teeth, we may safely infer—nay, more, we know positively, that these articles are to be reckoned among the many causes of consumption. It was well said by old Dr. Baynard, " In no one thing do people exhibit more ignorance than in the rearing of that noble creature, man."

Tobacco.—Tobacco, or *Nicotiana Tabacum*, belongs to the same natural order as *Atropa Belladonna*, and which is commonly known by the name of deadly night-shade, and the *Datura Stramonium*, or thorn-apple, both of which are among the most powerful and deadly of the acro-narcotic poisons. Hence we may infer that the constant use of this article must be capable of producing powerful effects on the living body. "From the habitual use of tobacco, in either of its forms—of snuff, cud, or cigar," says Professor Mussey, "the following symptoms may arise: a sense of weakness, sinking or pain at the pit of the stomach, dizziness or pain in the head, occasional dullness or temporary loss of sight, paleness and sallowness of the countenance, and sometimes swelling of the feet, enfeebled state of the voluntary muscles manifesting itself sometimes by tremulousness, weakness, squeaking, a hoarseness of the voice, rarely a loss of voice, disturbed sleep, starting from early slumbers with a sense of suffocation, or feeling of alarm, incubus or nightmare, epileptic or convulsive fits, confusion or weakness of the mental faculties, peevishness and irritability of temper, instability of purpose, seasons of great depressions of the spirits, long fits of unbroken melancholy and despondency, and, in some cases, entire and permanent mental derangement." "Tobacco," says Dr. Woodward, "is a powerful narcotic agent, and its use is very deleterious to the nervous system, producing tremors, vertigo, faintness, palpitation of the heart, derangement of the stomach, and other serious diseases. Judging from such authority, we may readily believe the statement of the great Dr. Rush, that he once lost a young man, seventeen years of age, of a pulmonary consumption, whose disorder was brought on by the intemperate use of cigars.

Hard water.—Hard water, which is generally abundant in the vicinity of mountains, is supposed to be productive of bronchocele (a peculiar tumor or swelling on the outside of the throat), which is to be regarded as a scrofulous disease. If this supposition is true, we may readily suppose that consumption, a kindred disease to scrofula—a scrofulous disease always, as some would have it—may also be caused in many cases by the use of hard water. Evidently this may be reckoned among one of the causes of consumption.

There appears to be a great amount of scrofula in the state of Vermont; and although this section of country is celebrated for its purity of air and exemption from marshes and malarious emanations, yet there appears to be a vast deal of scrofula and consumption in this state. There are now and then to be found springs of remarkable purity, but still the greater proportion of the springs, streams, and rivulets, which are to be found in such abundance in the Green Mountain country, are generally, so far as I have observed, very hard. All experience proves that the constant use of hard water in connection with other bad habits, is decidedly pernicious to the constitution. Hence there is reason to believe, as some physicians have done, that the use of water holding in solution large quantities of salts, such as lime, soda, etc., is to be regarded

7

often as a cause of scrofula, tubercles, and consumption. But some may here ask, if hard water is so deleterious to the constitution, why should it have been placed almost every where apparently for the use of man. To this I answer; first, an abundance of water falls from the clouds upon every man's house; and which, by the exercise of a little ingenuity, may be easily retained for use. Secondly, if we live upon the natural food of man, the farinacea and fruits, and avoid flesh meats and stimulants of whatever kind, thirst is seldom experienced at all. Living in this way, many persons have passed weeks, months, and some even years, without drinking or thirst. Evidently, however, water is man's natural drink, and if he exercises a moderate degree of ingenuity, there can be no excuse for his using water which is hard.

CHAPTER XVII.

Causes of consumption continued.—Suppression of habitual discharges.
—The depressing passions.—Striking examples given by Laennec.
—Sexual abuses.—Hæmorrhage from the lungs.—Inflammation of
the lungs.—Bronchitis and sore throat.—Opinions of various writers
on this subject.—Influenza.—Fevers.—Small-pox, scarletina, and
measles.—Their influence in developing tubercular disease.—Indigestion.

Suppression of habitual discharges.—A sudden suppression of the menstrual discharge, as by taking cold, has been known to develop latent consumption. Doubtless, too, this might, in connection with bad habits generally, become a prominent cause of bringing on the disease, even where a predisposition to it did not before exist. A sudden check of perspiration from exposure to cold, the checking of long-established cutaneous eruptions by stimulating washes, ointments, etc., and the healing up of old ulcers and fistulous openings may also develop this disease. These things act as a cause of consumption, more particularly where there is a predisposition to it.

The depressing passions.—"Mental depression," says Sir James Clark, "holds a very conspicuous place among those circumstances which diminish the powers of the system generally; and it often proves one of the most effectual determining causes of consumption. Disappointment of long-cherished hopes, slighted affections, loss of dearer relations, and reverses of fortune," continues this able writer, "often exert a powerful influence on persons predisposed to consumption, more particularly in the female sex."

Who is not familiar with the melancholy examples of consumption following close on the death of some near relative, some bosom friend, or disappointed and unrequited love?

Laennec records a striking example of the effect of the depressing passions, which example was ten years under his immediate observation. The account, as translated by Professor Sweetser, is as follows :

" There existed, during the time mentioned, at Paris, a recent religious community of women, who, on account of the extreme severity of their regulations, had obtained only a conditional toleration from the ecclesiastical authority. Their diet, though austere, yet did not exceed what the powers of nature could endure. But the rigor of their *religious* rules was productive of effects both melancholy and surprising. Their attention was not only habitually fixed on the most terrible truths of religion, but they were tried by all kinds of opposition to induce them, as soon as possible, to renounce entirely their own proper will. At the end of one or two months, the catamenia (menses) were suppressed ; and in one or two months more, phthisis was evident. They not being bound by vows, I urged them, on the first manifestation of the symptom of the malady, to quit the establishment ; and almost all who followed the advice were cured, though many of them had already exhibited evident signs of phthisis. During the ten years that I was physician to this household, I saw it renewed two or three times by the successive loss of all its members, with the exception of a very small number, composed principally of the superior, the grate-keeper, and the sisters who had the care of the garden, the kitchen, and the infirmary; and it is worthy of remark that these persons were those who had the most frequent distractions from their religious austerities, and that they frequently went out into the city on duties connected with the establishment."

It will, of course, be readily understood, that in all cases of this kind there are other causes besides that of mental depression merely, such as want of exercise, deficient ventilation, improper food, and the like, all of which aid in the production of the disease.

Sexual abuses.—If solitary vice, that one of the greatest of human curses, is sufficient, as is testified by Dr. Woodward, to cause idiocy, the most deplorable of all the forms of insanity, oftener than all other causes put together; if it is sufficient to cause an amount of depression of spirits, melancholy, dissatisfaction with life, and a waste of the strength of both body and mind to a most deplorable extent, as is often witnessed, we may well understand that this unseemly practice may often become a cause of consumption; nay, such must inevitably be the result. So, too, connubial excesses often develop this disease, as may be inferred from the fact that we often see the newly-married pass rapidly into hopeless decline. "I have seen many young men die of phthisis," says Dr. Elliotson, "a twelvemonth after their marriage, although they have shown no signs of it before."

Many a young man, too, in great cities—those hot-beds of pollution and of vice—has often, by a career of licentiousness, been brought early to the con-

sumptive's grave.　If a young man contract
most loathsome of all diseases, which arises from
tious habits, and if then, superadded to this, he
is generally the case, a course of medical treatment,
by which the system is saturated with mercury, iodine,
and like medicines, he may be very thankful if he does
not pass into a rapid consumption, or some other decline equally fatal.　But whatever may be the result,
he will find to a demonstration, which he will not soon
forget, that, "THE WAY OF THE TRANSGRESSOR IS HARD."

Hæmorrhage from the lungs.—People are generally
much alarmed at raising blood.　It is often difficult,
and many times impossible, to tell from whence the
blood comes; nor does this make any great difference.
Bleeding from the stomach indicates quite as bad a
state of things as bleeding from the lungs.　But I am
satisfied that pulmonary hæmorrhage, or the spitting
up of blood, is, in many instances, by no means so
unfavorable an omen as is generally supposed.　I have
known, in my practice, many who have bled from
the lungs, and have yet afterward recovered health.
I have been myself surprised, over and again, to see
with what facility persons have, by proper treatment,
outgrown difficulties of this kind.　Yet it should be
remembered that a bleeding from these important organs always indicates a wrong state of things, not only
in them, but in the system generally; and that, therefore, no pains should be spared in doing all in our
power to regain health, to fortify and invigorate the
general system.

Inflammation of the lungs.—That inflammation of
the lungs often precedes the development of consump-

tion, and that such inflammation may result in ulceration of these parts (which, although it is not really consumption, according to the modern acceptation of the term, but may yet cause death), is plainly true; but that such inflammation produces tubercles, there is no proof. But this has been the common doctrine among medical men. Inflammation of the lungs rarely affects both sides of the chest at a time, while consumption generally affects both lungs. Males are more subject to pulmonary inflammation, while females are more subject to consumption.

But although tuberculous matter is never the result of inflammation, it should be remembered that tuberculous subjects are more liable to inflammation than others. Hence, all persons who are predisposed to consumption, and such especially as those in whom we have reason to suspect that tubercles already exist, cannot be too careful in avoiding all causes of pulmonic inflammations. Such inflammation never fails to increase the mischief in those who are already laboring under tuberculous disease, and often serves to convert that which was before latent, and might in all probability have been kept in check for many years, into an active state of disease. Inflammation promotes the softening, or maturation, of tubercles, and thus hastens on their fearful work.

Bronchitis and sore throat.——Irritation and inflammation of the mucous membrane of the larynx, pharynx, and adjacent parts, or, in other words, the throat and trachea, or wind-pipe and bronchiæ (divisions of the trachea passing into the lungs), is supposed to be often the cause of tubercular consumption. Probably no affection whatever so commonly precedes it as throat and bronchial irritation. The pulmonary mucous membrane of tuberculous persons, is certainly very susceptible to the impressions of cold, moisture, vicissitudes of temperature, mechanical irritants conveyed into the air passages during respiration, and all those causes generally, which, in the nature of things, tend to produce irritation and inflammation of the part. Tubercles, too, often prove a source of bronchial mucous irritation, long before their presence can be detected by other symptoms. Repeated attacks of throat and bronchial inflammation, or the long-continued application of mechanical irritants to the mucous membrane of the air passages, it should be remembered, are very apt to prove exciting causes of consumption, especially when a constitutional predisposition to it exists.

Dr. Cullen regarded that consumption is liable to follow catarrh, or cold of the throat and lungs, only in constitutions already predisposed to it. "The beginning of consumption," he says, "so often resembles a catarrh, that the former might have been mistaken for the latter." Besides, to increase the fallacy, it often happens that the application of cold, which is the most frequent cause of catarrh, is also frequently the exciting cause of the cough which proves the beginning of consumption.

Louis, the celebrated French writer on pulmonary diseases, considers that the influence of pulmonary catarrh, in the production of consumption, is no better demonstrated than that of lung-fever, or inflammation of the lungs; and he affirms that females, who,

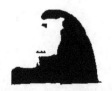

according to his observation, are more exposed to consumption than males, are less subject to pulmonary catarrh, or colds.

Andral holds, that if inflammation of the lining or mucous membranes, or the air passages, be followed by the production of pulmonary tubercles, it is necessary to admit a predisposition to them.

In view of this subject, then, it should be remarked that persons who are subject to the taking of cold in the throat and lungs, ought not to be alarmed at every trifling occurrence of the kind; although it is always better that such attacks should, as far as possible, be prevented. It should likewise always be remembered that in cases where a predisposition to pulmonary consumption is known to exist, a comparatively trifling cold may become a cause of exciting into action a fatal onset of the disease. At the same time, let no one blame himself when he knows he has been careful, and has avoided all possible causes of taking a cold, and yet finds such symptoms coming upon him; for consumption may be unavoidable in his case, and its beginning, in spite of all human means, must often be precisely like what appears the taking of an ordinary cold.

Influenza.—This disease, especially when epidemic, appears to sometimes hurry on to a final termination cases of chronic consumption. Those who have long labored under coughs, and other symptoms of pulmonary disease, have been frequently observed to die during this epidemic. Influenza may doubtless aid tubercular inflammatory action, and the softening or maturation of tubercles in the lungs; but that it can directly cause them, we have no reason to believe. The same prin-

7*

ciple holds good here, as in inflammation of the lungs, bronchitis, and the like.   It is not believed that any of these are sufficient, however, of themselves, to produce tubercles, although they may produce ulcerations of the lungs, and such as may lead to as fatal a termination as if tubercles existed.

Fevers.—Fevers, of whatever kind, whether continued, remittent, intermittent, bilious, or typhus, appear, generally, to hasten on the fearful work of consumption, where a strong predisposition to it exists, and in cases of inflammation of the lungs and air passages generally. We have no proof, however, that fever is a direct cause of tuberculous consumption.   It only operates by calling into action tubercles which already exist, or a tuberculous disposition of the individual.

The eruptive fevers, as small-pox, scarletina, and measles, appear often to develop this disease.   Hence, I may remark, too great care cannot be paid to the proper treatment of this disease.   The barbarous modes of stimulating such patients, keeping them in heated rooms, and under feather beds, in these diseases—modes which have been practiced to so great extent, for the last two centuries, cannot be too strongly deprecated.   Doubtless many a patient has been thrown into consumption by these means, and in which, if they had been treated by the cooling plan, which may be emphatically styled "nature's method," the terrible malady would have been, for a time at least, kept off.

Indigestion.—This has, by many, been regarded as one among the multiform causes of consumption.   It would, doubtless, be difficult, if not impossible, to prove that tubercles are ever caused by indigestion. But we know that bad food, bad air, and bad influences generally, are sufficient to generate tuberculous disease. As bad food, then. causes indigestion, we must regard this latter as bearing an important relation to tubercular consumption.

CHAPTER XVIII.

The causes of consumption concluded.—The different occupations.—Tables of M. Benoiston, made from observation in four of the Parisian hospitals, namely, L'Hotel Dieu, La Charite, La Pitie. and L'Hospice Cochin.—Results in occupations which expose the lungs to the action of an atmosphere loaded with vegetable dust.—Those which expose the lungs to the action of an atmosphere loaded with mineral particles.—Those which expose the lungs to the action of an atmosphere loaded with animal dust.—Occupations which expose the lungs to the action of an atmosphere loaded with hurtful vapors.—Those which expose the body, and particularly the feet, to the action of damp.—Occupations in which the muscles of the chest and arms are subject to a constant and fatiguing exercise.—Those in which the muscles of the arms and chest are subjected to constant motion while the body is maintained in a bent position.—Recapitulation of the more prominent causes of consumption.

Occupation as a cause of consumption.—We have but few well-arranged tables in medical literature that are calculated to give light on the important subject of the effect of different occupations in causing consumption. The most valuable ones which I have any where seen are those of M. Benoiston de Chateauneuf, drawn from observations in four of the Parisian hospitals, namely, L'Hotel Dieu, La Charite, La Pitie, and L'Hospice Cochin, during ten years, namely, from 1817 to 1827. For these tables I am indebted to a very accurate and able work—the Journal of Health, Philadelphia, 1832. page 91. The tables are as follows :

1. "*Occupations which expose the lungs to the action of an atmosphere loaded with vegetable dust:*

	Males.	Deaths.	Proport'n.
" Starch-makers, ...	98	1	1.02
Bakers, ...	2,702	56	2.07
Coalmen, ...	375	14	3.73
Forts de la Halle, ...	246	6	2.43
Rag-pickers, ...	590	5	0.84
Workers in cotton, ...	319	6	1.88
Spinners, ...	594	14	2.35

	Females.	Deaths.	Proport'n.
" Rag-pickers, ...	237	4	1.68
Workers in cotton, ...	882	24	2.72
Thread winders, ...	263	9	3.42
Spinners, ...	1,173	19	1.61

" Total number of males admitted of this class, 4924, of whom 102 died of consumption, or 2.07 per cent.

" Total number of females admitted of this class, 2555, of whom fifty-six died of consumption, or 2.19 per cent."

That rag-pickers should exhibit so low a degree of mortality as in the above table is certainly suprising, and if we are to judge from the results of these observations concerning the effects of " factory life," as it is called in this country, it is by no means so unhealthful as many suppose it to be.

2. "*Occupations which expose the lungs to the action of an atmosphere loaded with mineral particles:*

	Males.	Deaths.	Proport'n.
" Stone-quarriers, ...	887	13	1.46
Masons and laborers, ...	4,071	90	2,22
Stone-cutters, ...	162	2	1.25
Plasterers, ...	158	4	2.53
Lapidaries, ...:.........	551	5	0.90

"Total number of this class admitted, 5829, all males, of whom 114 died of consumption, 1.95 per cent."

According to this table, stone-cutters, with the exception of lapidaries (dealers in precious stones), were the least subject to consumption. It has been supposed by many that this occupation is necessarily one of the most injurious of all to the lungs. The contact with dust and fine particles of stone to which the laborer is constantly subjected, has been regarded as very detrimental to the health of the lungs. Stone-quarriers also come, to a certain extent, under this head; that is, they too are much exposed to the di·· and dust arising from the cutting and blasting of stones, and yet their proportion of deaths is very small.

Comparing this table with the last, we find the per centage of deaths a little less in the latter. In connection, it is to be observed, that the occupations of the last are more out-door and active in their nature than the former.

3. "*Occupations which expose the lungs to the action of an atmosphere loaded with animal dust :*

	Males.	Deaths.	Proport'n.
" Brush-makers,	283	10	3.53
Carders of wool and hair,	129	4	3.10
Hatters,	983	47	4.78
Feather workers,	39	3	7.69

	Females.	Deaths.	Proport'n.
" Brush-makers,	103	8	7.76
Carders of wool and hair,	451	11	2.43
Hatters,	130	1	0.55
Feather workers,	61	7	11.47

"Total number of males admitted of this class, 1434, of whom sixty-four died of consumption, or 4.46 per cent.

"Total number of females admitted of this class, 795, of whom twenty-seven died of consumption, or 3.39 per cent."

Comparing this last table with the next preceding, it would seem that in-door workers have a poorer chance in reference to consumption than such as are engaged in active out-door pursuits.

The per centage of deaths among females according to this table is less than that of males, which is supposed to be different from the general rule.

4. "*Occupations which expose the lungs to the action of an atmosphere loaded with hurtful vapors :*

	Males.	Deaths.	Propor'tn.
"Gilders,.............................	545	29	5.32
Painters and ornamenters,........	2,160	47	2.17
Fumigators, ...	389	13	3.34

	Females.	Deaths.	Propor'tn.
"Gilders, ...	285	16	5.61

"Total number of males admitted of this class, 3094, of whom eighty-nine died of consumption, or 2.87 per cent.

"Total number of females admitted of this class, 285, of whom sixteen died of consumption, or 5.61 per cent."

According to this table, painters and ornamenters have a much better chance, in regard to consumption, than many of those of the other occupations.

5. "*Occupations which expose the body, and particularly the feet, to the action of damp :* .

	Males.	Deaths.	Proport'n.
"Bleachers,.....................	218	4	1.83

	Females.	Deaths.	Proport'n.
"Bleachers, ...	2,775	125	4.50."

It is to be observed, in reference to this table, that males, who generally dress their feet and lower extremities with greater care, or more perfectly than females, have a much lower proportion of deaths in those occupations where these parts are much exposed to cold and damp. These results afford, I conceive, an important practical lesson on this point.

6. "*Occupations in which the muscles of the chest and arms are subjected to a constant and fatiguing exercise :*

	Males.	Deaths.	Proport'n.
"Weavers,...................	935	20	2.13
Gauze-makers, ...	251	8	3.18
Carpenters, ...	286	4	1.49
Joiners,....................	1,716	53	3.08
Blacksmiths, etc., ...	214	2	0.93
Locksmiths, ...	668	5	0,74
Water-carriers, ...	373	9	2.41
Stone-sawyers, etc., ...	702	8	1.13

	Females.	Deaths.	Proport'n.
"Weavers, ...	163	3	1.84
Gauze-makers, ...	253	8	3.16

"Total number of males admitted of this class, 5127, of whom 109 died of consumption, or 2.12 per cent.

"Total number of females admitted of this class, 416, of whom eleven died of consumption, or 2.64 per cent."

We see, in reference to this table, that carpenters have a much lower average of deaths from consumption than joiners.   The latter do the in-door work of buildings, the former the out-door work, which is certainly, in many respects, the more healthy occupation of the two.   It is remarkable, too, that blacksmiths and locksmiths, the trades of both of which are very laborious, while at the same time both classes are subject much to dirt, dust, iron filings, and the like, have yet a very low average of deaths from this disease. Stone-sawyers, too, who work, for the most part, out doors, and are yet much subject to particles of dust from the stone, have a very low average.   This table, on the whole, speaks well for hard and fatiguing labor, in the open air and light.

7. *" Occupations in which the muscles of the chest and arms are subjected to constant motion, while the body is maintained in a bent position :*

	Males.	Deaths.	Proport'n.
" Scriveners,	908	43	4.73
Jewelers,	715	46	6.43
Tailors,	1,048	49	4.67
Shoemakers,	1,818	78	4.29
Fringe and lace-makers,	426	20	4.69
Cutters of crystal,	244	15	6.14
Polishers,	270	12	4.44
	Females.	Deaths.	Proport'n.
" Jewelers,	39	4	13.33
Tailors,	1,069	49	4.58
Fringe and lace-makers,	534	25	4.68
Polishers,	548	21	3.83
Shoe-binders,	397	22	5.54
Embroiderers,	593	51	8.60
Seamstresses,	5,392	296	5.48

	Females.	Deaths.	Proport'n.
Flower-makers,	357	31	8.68
Bone-lace makers,	258	16	6.20
Glove-makers,	402	26	6.46
Menders,	540	33	6.11

"Total number of males admitted of this class, 5429, of whom 263 died of consumption, or 4.84 per cent.

"Total number of females admitted of this class, 10,129, of whom 574 died of consumption, or 5.66 per cent.

"Total number of males of all the foregoing classes admitted, 26,055, of whom 745 died of consumption, or 2.85 per cent.

"Total number of females 16,955; deaths 809, or 4.77 per cent.

"Total number of individuals, of both sexes, 43,010, among whom the deaths by consumption were 1554.

"Proportion of deaths by consumption to whole number of patients who were admitted, 3.61 per cent."

We see, according to the last table of M. Benoiston, the injurious effects of those occupations which confine persons within doors, and for the most part in a bent and sitting posture. The averages, among all these occupations, it will be seen, are higher than those of most others. Habitual stooping of the body is, beyond doubt, one of the greatest of all causes of consumption.

It must be admitted that all such tables as the above, even when drawn up by the most careful and accurate observers, are liable to more or less imperfections. It is only by observing a considerable number of them that we can arrive at an approximation of truth. But all such tables are, on the whole, very valuable and interesting.

"There are certain occupations," says Dr. Clark, "which are generally considered unfavorable to the occurrence of consumption : those of seamen, butchers, and tanners hold the first rank. Various reasons have been adduced to account for this exemption. I have no doubt that it is chiefly attributable to the free and regular exercise in the open air which they enjoy."

To conclude, then, on the causes of consumption, as shown in the foregoing chapters, the more prominent may be stated as the following :

1. Hereditary predisposition.
2. Impure air.
3. Want of light.
4. Insufficient food.
5. Excess of food.
6. Deficient bodily exercise.
7. Excessive labor.
8. Over-exertion of the lungs.
9. Excessive mental labor.
10. Improper clothing.
11. Want of cleanliness.
12. Spirituous drinks.
13. Mercury.
14. Abuse of medicines generally.
15. Tobacco.
16. Tea and coffee.
17. Hard water.
18. Suppression of the natural discharges.

19. The depressing passions.
20. Sexual abuses.
21. Hæmorrhage from the lungs.
22. Inflammation of the lungs.
23. Bronchitis and sore throat.
24. Influenza.
25. Fevers.
26. Dyspepsy.

And lastly, all causes, and all occupations which tend to deteriorate the general health

CHAPTER XIX.

Hæmorrhage from the lungs.—This often exists as one of the earliest symptoms of tubercular consumption.—It is a symptom not always dangerous, but one that demands special attention. Females are most subject to it.—Opinions of Louis and Dr. Sweetser.—Age at which pulmonary hæmorrhage most frequently occurs.—This affection is not necessarily associated with a consumptive habit.—Nature of the affection.—Means of knowing it.—Bright red or arterial blood usually comes from the lungs, and dark or venous blood from the stomach.—Symptoms that immediately precede bleeding from the lungs.—Effects of pulmonary hæmorrhage on the system. —Causes of this affection.—It appears sometimes to be a friendly disease.—Its treatment.—Injurious effects of fear.—Pulmonary hæmorrhage should be treated on the same principles as an inflammation.—Dr. Elliotson's method.—Bleeding and cold on the chest. —Blisters.—The general principles and the particulars of the treatment stated.—The true methods of avoiding a recurrence of this disease.

As hæmorrhage from the lungs is often associated with consumption, and in many cases exists as one of its earliest symptoms, it will be proper to enter somewhat into detail concerning it. I have remarked elsewhere that persons are generally much alarmed at symptoms of this kind, and more so, often, than there is any need of. I have also remarked, that in many instances persons have, by proper treatment, outgrown these difficulties. Still, however, it must be confessed that pulmonary hæmorrhage ought always to be looked upon as a serious matter, and one that demands special attention on the part, both of the patient and the physician.

Females more subject than than males to pulmonary hæmorrhage.—The observations of various writers go to prove that this affection is more common among females than males. According to Louis, the proportion is as three to two. Professor Sweetser is of the opinion, also, that the observations of medical men in this country, in relation to pulmonary hæmorrhage, would lead to like results with those of the French physicians. Hæmorrhage from the stomach is doubtless much more frequent also in women than men.

Age at which it occurs.—Pulmonary hæmorrhage will be found to occur oftenest at that period of life when the system is most liable to consumption. Thus it will seldom be observed before fourteen or fifteen years of age, or, in other words, before puberty, and seldom after forty. Between eighteen and thirty-five, may be stated as the period in which persons are most liable to this affection. It occurs oftenest at that period during which the chest expands, and we spread, as is said. "The first part of life," says Dr. Elliotson, "is disposed to hæmorrhage from the nostrils; the second, to hæmorrhage from the lungs; and the third, to hæmorrhage from the abdomen."

Not necessarily associated with a consumptive habit.—We not unfrequently see persons who have been liable to considerable spitting of blood, and without any apparent injury to health, during many years of their life. Dr. Heberden gives an account of a woman at seventy, in good condition, who, for fifty years, had never been free from this symptom above two years together. Pulmonary hæmorrhage may happen in

persons in whom there are no reasons for suspecting
tubercles, and who appear to be, in no respect, of a
consumptive habit.

Nature of the affection. —The bleeding is supposed
to proceed oftenest from the air passages, or from the
air-cells of the lungs. Probably the popular notion
that hæmorrhage from the lungs is owing to the rupture of a blood-vessel, seldom holds true. Such, it'is
true, may sometimes be the case, as in the advanced
stages of consumption, when there has been great destruction of the substance of the lungs. But in the
greater number of cases the hæmorrhage arises simply
from the affusion of blood from the mucous membrane
within the lungs. This hæmorrhage being often, then,
simply an affusion or oozing of blood from the mucous
membrane, and not from a ruptured blood-vessel, we
may readily understand why it is that we so often
succeed in curing it.

Signs by which it is known.—The principal difficulty is to distinguish between it and bleeding from
the stomach. The latter may be more commonly
known by the discharges, consisting of black blood.
The blood is either discharged from the veins of the
stomach, or it lies in the stomach so long after it escapes from the vessels, that it acquires a venous hue.
From the one cause or from the other, blood, when
discharged upward from the stomach, is generally
black ; and has, also, generally lain there long enough
to be coagulated—it is in clots, larger or smaller.
Frequently, too, it passes through the pylorus, and is
seen in the discharges from the bowels. Besides that,
it frequently comes up with the food, and other contents

of the stomach ; and, when it does not, still it comes up with sickness and nausea, if not with downright vomiting. We know that people may have a discharge from the stomach without vomiting ; sometimes a quantity of fluid comes to the mouth, and even portions of food, without any retching ; and so it is with the blood. Occasionally, however, it comes up with decided vomiting. There is frequently a great uneasiness about the præcordia, and a fullness about the liver and stomach. These symptoms are absent in hæmorrhage from the lungs. The blood, here, is florid ; and instead of being mixed with food, it is frothy, and is necessarily mixed with air, in consequence of the parts from which it comes containing always a large quantity of it. These parts will not allow it to stay so long as in the stomach ; and it generally comes up as soon as it is poured into the passages, and it is therefore seldom coagulated. Occasionally, however, there is a little coagulum ; for it will sometimes lie sufficiently long to become solid and black, before it comes up. In addition to this, we have pectoral symptoms in hæmorrhage from the lungs ; instead of nausea and vomiting, there is a " stitch in the side, a little cough, and a tickling in the throat. On listening to the chest, when the blood is in the air passages, we hear sibilous and sonorous rattles."

The signs immediately preceding the flow of blood, may be distinct and strongly marked, or scarcely appreciable. Sometimes it may happen without any premonition, but, as a general fact, there may be noticed some febrile excitement, and especially signs of preternatural determination of blood to the lungs. Among the more threatening symptoms, there is sense of weight, weight and oppression about the chest, and more or less embarrassment of breathing, especially if any effort be made. There is, also, a sense of heat within the chest, particularly in the breast bone. Lassitude, paleness, and coldness of the skin, shivering and coldness of the extremities, all of which are sometimes felt, indicate that the blood is pressing inward too much upon the lungs. The patient experiences, often, an unusual desire for fresh air, immediately preceding the attack. And some persons, subject to pulmonary hæmorrhage, have had warning of a tendency to an attack, by their being obliged, contrary to their usual custom, to sleep with a window open, otherwise breathing would become distressing, and sleep disturbed.

Quantity of blood emitted.—Sometimes the discharges may hardly be said to consist of blood at all, the common mucous of the air passages being merely tinged with it. These symptoms may continue for several days, or even weeks, and then cease; or they may be followed by a considerable gush of pure blood.

Often the hæmorrhage seems at once to relieve the over-loaded vessels and then ceases, to return again at longer or shorter intervals; or, as happens in some cases, disappears forever.

The hæmorrhage will be found varying from several mouthfuls to a teacup full; but it is difficult in many cases to determine the precise amount. There is often so much alarm at the moment, that persons are very apt to over-state the quantity. Bright blood,

8

it should be remembered, makes a great show. It always appears more than it really is.

Effects on the system.—The effects of pulmonary hæmorrhage are often trifling; and it not unfrequently, as before remarked, brings relief to the system. At other times, the individual is able very soon, almost at once, to go about his ordinary avocation. At other times the system becomes much prostrated, so that the patient may be an invalid for weeks. At other times, in the advanced stages of consumption, it may be the means of quickly closing the death-scene.

Causes.—This disease sometimes occurs when we can scarcely attribute it to any particular cause; and sometimes in the presence of great strength of general system, and apparently good health. Cold, and variable conditions of the atmosphere, may act as an exciting cause. Diminution of atmospheric pressure, as on the ascent of very elevated mountains, is said to have caused it. Irritating substances breathed into the lungs, intemperance in the use of spirituous liquors, excess of food, and whatever occasions plethora of the system, violent exercise of the body, and especially over-exertion of the lungs, as in playing on instruments, or in long-continued reading and speaking, fear, and all strong mental emotions, may cause Broussais relates an instance where a lady, sitting the grass, felt a living frog fall into her bosom from the claws of a bird of prey, and was instantly seized with so copious a bleeding from the lungs that she survived but a few minutes. Long-continued and excessive laughing has also been known to cause it. A fall, or a blow upon the chest, may also bring on pulmonary hæmorrhage. A sudden suppression of perspiration, checking of cutaneous eruptions, and of any habitual discharge whatever, may also bring on this affection.

Sometimes friendly to the system.—We know that bleeding from the nose not unfrequently cures headache and oppression of the brain. We know, too, that bleeding from the bowels in fevers, and some other diseases, appears sometimes to be nature's method of effecting a cure. So, also, we may conclude that bleeding from the lungs is, in some instances at least, a natural effort of the system. Despite of the fright it generally causes, it often relieves oppression and embarrassment in the lungs, and doubtless does the individual decided good.

Treatment.—I have said that many persons recover from bleeding at the lungs, even from severe attacks. Dr. Elliotson tells us, that he has known many persons who had expectorated blood fifteen or twenty years before he wrote on the subject, and who were at the time well. I can myself call to mind a number of persons who have had pulmonary hæmorrhage over and over again, so much so at times, as to prostrate the system very much; and although this happened a number of years since, those persons are now comparatively well; better, perhaps, than ever before in their lives, and more hardy and enduring than people generally are. These facts should give us courage in the treatment of this affection, and, at the same time, teach individuals subject to it the important lesson that they should not become alarmed and frightened almost out of their senses at every little oozing of blood from these parts; and yet I would not have this advice construed into an excuse for carelessness in regard to the means and necessity of observing all good rules of health, so that the individual may, as far as possible, avoid al. such attacks.

The treatment of the slighter forms of pulmonary hæmorrhage, is to be comprehended by a reference to all those rules and habits generally, the observance of which tend to fortify and invigorate the general health; and I shall here but repeat, that I assert that people generally are far more frightened than there is any occasion for, in attacks of this kind; yet at the same time all who have hæmorrhage from the lungs, however slight, should spare no pains, however great, in order to establish a permanent state of general health. When an individual has lost this best of all earthly blessings, and is made to quail under the influence of an incurable disorder, what would he not give if he could again be made well? All the wealth of the city of New York, the wealth of the Indies, yea, more, the wealth of the whole world combined, would be as nothing in the balance when compared with that most important matter, the restoration of health. May I not hope, then, that some at least will heed my admonition. In the alarming cases of this disorder, prompt and decided measures are often necessary. Such attacks, too, often come on suddenly, so that even perhaps at the most critical time the presence of the physician cannot be had. Hence the necessity for people to learn how to do for themselves.

It should be remembered that wherever there is hæmorrhage—no matter in what part of the living

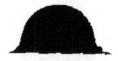

system—too much heat exists; hence all judicious physicians treat hæmorrhage on the principle of *inflammation*, singular as the practice may appear. I will here remark, that as much as I deprecate bleeding, as a general thing, I have no doubt persons have often been saved in hæmorrhage, by the artificial abstraction of blood; but I maintain that there is yet a better means, one which is more effectual in bringing about the desired object, and at the same time leaves the blood, "in which is the life thereof," within the system, so that recovery may be much more speedy in the end.

"Bleed in the arm freely," says Dr. Elliotson, "and set the patient upright, and keep him so, in order to make him feel as faint as possible;" and then adds, with his good sense, "it is safe to apply ice to the front of the chest; and this, I think, should always be done. There can be no impropriety in it. As soon as we have bled, until ice can be procured, we should throw cold water on the chest, and endeavor to produce a contraction of the end of the vessel—in the same way as we proceed in the case of the womb. But generally the bleeding soon stops; for a patient seldom dies of pulmonary hæmorrhage at the time. Bleeding at the arm, throwing open the windows and doors, and taking the clothes off the chest, answers very well. The patient should not be allowed to move. He should be made easy and comfortable; but he should not be allowed to move, or speak. I have often made persons persevere, for a fortnight together, after dangerous hæmorrhage, making them write for whatever was wanted. It is proper to starve the patient; to give him nothing but plain water, milk and water, lemonade, or things of that description; and it is surprising how patients, in this disease, bear cold."

This quotation gives, in short terms, the sum and substance of the orthodox treatment in this disease— a treatment, too, which is conducted on physiological principles, although the means of the treatment are not always such as I would agree with.

Acetate of lead, the extract of tannin, or tannic acid, and a great variety of other remedies, are sometimes also resorted to, in this affection. Dr. Rush had a favorite remedy, which he used to check the bleeding, and which may now, in this country, be considered a popular remedy—namely, common salt, taken in a dose of a teaspoonful, every few hours, till the hæmorrhage abates. This article, although so common and so much used, is a powerful drug, when taken in such quantities. I should be unwilling to take it myself; but it is doubtless as good as any other of the drug remedies that are given with the view of arresting the flow of blood.

Blisters on the chest have been resorted to, and I am not prepared to say that these do not often do good. Dr. Elliotson regards them as good in the latter part of the treatment; but the application of cold by means of ice, he regards as being better. But I should myself prefer cold wet cloths even to ice. I think ice is, in general, too severe a measure; that is, more severe than is necessary. By the use of cold wet cloths, we may abstract the same amount of heat from the part, by continuing the application a little longer, often rubbing it, and thus not do so great violence to the system. I have reason to believe that, in all cases where ice is used, as upon the scalp, chest, and whatever part, the cold cloths are better ; and we can always get cold well-water, but not so with ice. There is a tendency with practitioners generally, I think, and also with the people, to desire a remedy that is more powerful than is natural, or necessary ; and thus, by overdoing a good thing, I am confident, harm is sometimes done.

The coldness of the extremities and surface, often experienced in severe hæmorrhage from the lungs, symptoms which show that the blood is pressing inward too much upon the affected part, teaches us to resort to means which will tend to bring the blood back again more toward the surface and extreme parts of the system. And one of the best possible means for accomplishing this, probably *the* best, is to wash the surface smartly with the palms of the wet hand. Wet friction upon the skin is certainly a very admirable means of exciting cutaneous circulation ; at the same time, it refreshes the general system, cools the circulation, and supports the patient's strength.

It is well, I am convinced, in these cases—especially when the feet are cold, to put them into warm water ; at the same time the washing over of the general surface may be followed up.

The parts of the treatment, then, in severe hæmorrhage from the lungs, may be stated like the following :

1. To make cold applications to the chest by means of cloths wet in cold water, or by pounded ice or snow

in their season, so as effectually to cool the mass of the circulation ;

2. To practice wet friction over the general system ;

3. To take frequently small quantities of water internally, and even pieces of ice, where this is desired ;

4. To cool the back of the head, the neck and spine, generally ; and,

5. To keep the feet in warm water, and make other warm applications to them when necessary.

After the hæmorrhage has been arrested by the means of thus effectually cooling the blood and regulating the circulation, the general principles of good nursing, such as apply in all serious diseases, it will be understood, are to be observed. And here I will remark, that quite as much depends upon how the nursing is performed, as upon what the medical adviser does. I will remark, also, that Dr. Elliotson of London —as high authority as can be quoted in the old-school practice, tells us—and he has had great experience in these things, that it is surprising how patients in this disease bear cold. " I know not a single instance of a person suffering inflammation of the chest from all this exposure," he remarks, "notwithstanding that in other circumstances he would, in all probability, have suffered severely."

Thus, I think, it will appear plain that any individual of good understanding, provided the patient have confidence in simple means, may safely and efficiently treat this often serious malady. If I were myself attacked by this formidable affection, I should most certainly resort to the means I have here described—in short, to the cool or cold water plan, by far in preference to that of any other; and this, not because I have advocated it, and recommended it to others heretofore,.*but simply because I believe it to be the best.* I hope to have no other hobby than that of the most earnest love for truth.

CHAPTER XX.

The treatment of consumption continued.—Cough.—Opium and antimony.—Washing the surface with pure water.—Fasting.—Evils of
over-eating.—Saccharine matter.—Difficulty of respiration.—How
treated.—The expectoration.—Diet and water-drinking as a means
of modifying it.—Perspiration.—The great power of water to pre
vent the debilitating sweats of consumption.—Evils of feather beds
in causing hectic night sweats.—Airing the bedclothes in the night,
and exposing the surface of the body to the atmosphere a useful
means.—Dr. Marshall Hall's remarks on sponging the surface with
salt water.—The fresh is still better.—The hectic fever.—Means
of modifying it.—The pulse.—Means of modifying it.—Exercise
good, but should not be too violent.—Diarrhœa.—Palliative treatment to be used.—Pains of the chest.—Wet fomentations better
than blisters.—Care to be exercised in making the wet applications.
—Debility in consumption.—How to modify it.—The true principles on which consumption is to be treated.—Remarks of Drs. Billing and Elliotson.—Bathing and exercise the greatest of all known
means for preventing this disease.

Cough.—This being a troublesome symptom, a great
variety of remedial means have, from time immemorial, been resorted to with the hope of benefiting it.
Our newspapers are filled with advertisements of cough
mixtures, cough candy, and the like.

Opium will often relieve a cough, although it does
not always produce this effect. Whatever good it
may do, in preventing this symptom. is accomplished
only by its power of lessening the general vitality of
the system. It must necessarily do harm in the end.

Antimony, in some of its preparations, combined either with or without opium, is also much used in coughs. This is also a most pernicious drug.

One of the best palliative means for cough, when consumption has not proceeded to a great extent, is to make the body naked, and wash the surface with pure water, especially the throat and chest. Even washing the feet will often relieve a troublesome cough. Walking or riding in the open air is also good. Omitting a meal, especially at night, will many times make a material difference in this symptom. The sipping frequently of pure soft water, when a cough is troublesome, is also a most excellent means. There is more or less feverishness in the blood always, when troublesome coughing occurs, and hence it is that washing the surface, and drinking water, that is, cooling the mass of the circulation somewhat, is good in these cases.

Over-eating, it should be remembered, always aggravates a cough. In some cases of bronchitis, and perhaps in the early stages of consumption, where cough is troublesome at night, so as to keep the patient awake, a little honey, or other saccharine matter, taken into the stomach, appears to do good. I know that, in my own person, I nave at times had a very troublesome cough, which would keep me awake for hours sometimes in the night; and I found that by taking a small piece of sugar into the mouth, the lungs became soothed and quiet, so that I very soon feil asleep. Now the way in which this remedy operates is by mere sympathy. The saccharine substance passes into the stomach; in doing so, however, it comes in contact with the epiglottis, and so, by sympathy, operates upon the wind-pipe, where the irritation exists. We know that getting a piece of sugar, or any other substance, "the wrong way," would only make us cough the harder. But I recommend, in this matter, that patients be very careful how they indulge in sweets, with the hope of relieving cough. Saccharine matter is always hard of digestion, and is necessarily very apt to derange the stomach. It is possible that it does good in some instances, as I have mentioned, by procuring sleep, when one would otherwise be kept awake; but great care is necessary to be observed, or more harm than good will be the result of this practice.

The difficulty of breathing, which often attends lung complaints, may be greatly modified and relieved by the washings and wet hand frictions, such as I have recommended for cough. Here, too, we must be careful in diet, and also in regard to pure air. The same general rules which apply in cough, apply also to this symptom.

The *expectoration* may be greatly modified in its character by diet, and especially by the drinking of pure soft water. If the food is simple and unstimulating, the expectoration will be less.

Perspiration.—The power of water to promote the strength of the living tissue, is nowhere more strikingly exemplified than in the treatment of hectic night sweats. With every thing besides well managed, it would seem that these debilitating night sweats can be effectually checked, to the very last. Often have I known persons, who have sweltered for weeks and months, nightly, with perspiration, in whom it was checked altogether by the simple effect of cold water, and wet frictions upon the surface. Nor would I have the water applied very cold ; only of such temperature as the patient can bear, that is, can get comfortably warm after. In proportion as these night sweats are checked by water, is the strength supported, the health made more comfortable in every respect, and, to all appearance, life materially prolonged. These washings may be practiced two or three times daily, with the view of invigorating the surface. Pure fresh water—the purer and softer the better—should be used.

Feather beds often do a great deal of harm in causing night sweats. Perhaps it would be impossible for all persons, when they become much emaciated, so that the bones almost protrude through the skin, to lie upon hard beds. I would not say that those poor sufferers should never lie upon feather beds. I would gladly do any thing, if it were not positively and decidedly prejudicial, to promote the comfort, in any degree, however small, of those suffering patients ; but I would advise that great care be taken in regard to the bedding. Avoid feathers, both for the bed and pillow, as far as possible.

Have the bed clothing well aired, and the cleaner the better. The patient, too, should have the coolest and most airy room in the house. The bed should be placed as near the middle of it as may be ; never have the head away in the corner of the room, for in that situation the air must be breathed over more than in the former. Would that all consumptive patients

might be placed in comfortable and independent circumstances, in all that pertains to this life.

Getting up in the night-time and airing the bed,
and walking about in the air of the room, if not too
cold, will help to prevent the night perspirations.
Going to a fresh bed will also often check them.

Sponging the surface with salt water.—Dr. Mar-
shal Hall speaks strongly in favor of sponging the
surface with a solution consisting of one ounce of
common salt dissolved in one pint of water. With
this the patient is to sponge the whole surface, using
it as he recommends, warm in winter, tepid in spring
and autumn, and cold in summer. But what temperature is meant by the terms "warm," "tepid," and
"cold?" This is an important matter which does not
appear. As for the salt, it had better be omitted,
because it injures the skin. If water is taken warm,
that is about the temperature of the blood, it is very
liable to debilitate the system, and to give the patient
a cold. I regard that it is better to take it a little
cooler. Dr. Marshall Hall is correct, however, when
he recommends the repetition of the morning sponging "*as the most effectual remedy for the colli-
quative perspirations of tuberculous patients* in the
night, or early part of the morning." Let the patient,
if he can, remove to another bed after this sponging,
and he will be more apt to pass the remainder of
an otherwise wearisome night in refreshing sleep.
Changing the night clothes and sheets is also serviceable. So trifling a matter, as going from one bed to
another, changing the clothes, or even getting up and
airing the bed, at the same time exposing the surface

of the body to the atmosphere for a few minutes, will often help much to keep back this perspiration, and thus aid in procuring good sleep.

But the washing the surface when it is warm, two or three times in the twenty-four hours, with water cool and yet not too cold, that is, not so cold as to shock or over-chill the system, is, as before remarked, the great and sovereign remedy for preventing the night sweats of consumption, as well also as that of all other debilitating diseases. But this effect is produced by the tonic or strengthening effect of cold water and friction upon the skin. Not only is the skin strengthened by this practice, but the whole system. Sleep, too, is thus made better; and this aids also in keeping up the general strength. Thus one good influence aids another.

Hectic fever.—Nature teaches us, most unequivocally, as to what is the greatest as well as the most abundant of all febrifuges. All other remedies than pure water and fresh air dwindle into comparative insignificance when compared with water. As soon as the consumptive patient begins to feel the heat coming into the feet and hands, let him at once commence washing these parts. He need not take the water extremely cold, but washing freely the face, hands, and arms often accomplishes wonders in keeping down this symptom.

Heat, it should be remembered, takes away the strength rapidly. It is heat, too, that causes delirium in fevers; and if this is properly attended to by the cooling plan, I think that symptom can never occur in this disease. In proportion as the heat is kept down, the strength will be supported, and the mind rendered more clear. Perseverance in this method also aids in keeping off debilitating sweats. Sweating comes on in proportion to the amount of feverishness, as a general thing; hence to remedy the one is equivalent to preventing the other.

The pulse.——This is always more or less accelerated and feeble in consumption. It varies in different individuals and at different periods of the disease. It varies also during each day, rising in proportion to the general feverishness, and most toward night, as a general thing. After consumption has fairly commenced, the pulse may be said to range from ninety to a hundred beats per minute, and upward. It is small and feeble, and such as indicates great debility of the system.

The *cooling treatment* has a great influence in regulating the velocity of the circulation. Any thing which tends to prevent the feverishness, acts in bringing the pulse to a more natural standard. But in order to remedy this symptom fully and permanently, the system must be capable of being so invigorated as to prevent all general and unnatural debility. So long as the system remains enfeebled, the pulse is liable to become too quick.

Exercise is an invaluable means in consumption; but if this be too great, the heart is made to beat too quick, and the general circulation is accelerated. It is important, therefore, that consumptive persons should not exercise too much; and one of the methods of knowing how to graduate the exercise, is by observing the frequency of the pulse.

Over-heated rooms always exercise a pernicious influence on the circulation. It is common for consumptive patients to be kept in rooms that are much warmed. An individual remaining constantly in heated air cannot at all judge properly by his feelings as to what temperature is best suited to his case. Indeed, the more the air is heated above a certain standard, the more the patient suffers from cold, and, as a consequence, the more fire is desired. A few weeks since, being in the state of Vermont, I was taken to see a young man far gone in consumption, who was yet, however, able to sit up, and even to ride out. It was on Sunday, when the family were at home, and they were all seated in a room heated by a stove. As I entered it, the air appeared most oppressively hot, and could not have been less than 80° Fahr., I think, when at the same time the weather was decidedly cool. The young man complained of great debility, and his pulse had risen (it was in the afternoon) to 110 beats per minute. I directed the door to be opened a little way, and after sitting about half an hour, and when the air had become a good deal cooled, I again examined the pulse. It had fallen ten beats per minute; and this was solely attributable to the change made by opening the door. Imagine that this young man had gone on from day to day in thus accelerating the velocity of the heart's action by the over-heated air of his room. We can readily imagine how much faster his life would have been worn out.

The *thirst* is not generally a troublesome symptom in pulmonary disease. It occurs, however, not unfrequently to some extent. The principles of treating it in whatever disease are the same. The free use of fruits, as a part of the regular meals, aids much in keeping off both feverishness and thirst.

The *diarrhœa* occurs generally in proportion to the debility present; hence any thing which tends to a betterment of the health and strength, will aid in keeping off this symptom. It arises in consequence of ulceration of the bowels; hence a radical cure can seldom be effected. I would have persons distinguish, however, that during the progress of consumption, they may very easily, at times, have other forms of diarrhœa than that which attends its latter stages, so that they should not become alarmed at every little attack of the kind they may experience.

As a palliative means to be used in the fatal diarrhœa which occurs toward the last of consumption, pretty copious injections of lukewarm or tepid water into the bowels, will be found a most excellent means. It serves to soothe the patient, and at the same time supports his strength. Have a good instrument, and resort to the internal rinsing at every time when the bowels act unnaturally. Use it either just before, or after, or both. Be the diarrhœa of whatever kind, this is a most excellent remedy.

Pains in the chest.—Shall we put on blisters or make sores with an ointment of tartar emetic, or some other escharotic, for pains in the chest? Such will certainly relieve them; but I think the application of mustard would be a preferable means to any of these and safer, certainly.

All of these means, I firmly believe, do almost always more harm than good in the end, especially the former articles ; besides, I believe there is a more effectual way than either of these, and that is, the application of wet compresses over the part where the pain exists, and over the whole chest, if necessary. We wring wet towels tolerably dry out of cold water, lay these upon the chest, over these dry flannels, or other materials enough to insure a tolerable degree of warmth. Some have worn wet jackets over the whole chest—one, two, or three thicknesses, and then dry ones enough to insure the proper degree of warmth In hot climates and hot seasons any where, these applications are liable to become almost immediately too warm, and so to debilitate the system. At such times, the frequent washings of the chest with the wet hand will be found preferable. This may be done repeatedly during the day. Any one who is timid in regard to these applications—and all should be careful in their use—can commence with a simple application, a single napkin, or the like, at first ; place it over the most painful part, and watch its effects ; and if it does well, a larger application may be made, and so on to any extent desired.

If there is already extensive ulceration, these applications must be made cautiously. The system must not be too much chilled in such cases, if so, harm will be done. With a little exercise, the patient's feelings will be a sufficient guide in this matter. Let him remember, however, if his case be a bad one, that when there is so much prejudice as now exists in the world against the use of cold water, and so much ignorance of its effects, if he wear the wet cloths, and is perfectly sensible that they do him good, and if

he yet is doomed to get worse, in consequence of the
incurability of his case, there will not be wanting
those among his friends who will be ready enough to
tell him that these water applications have caused
his death.   With the great and all-pervading ignorance that exists concerning the use of this safest
of all nature's remedies, people would a great deal
rather be bled, blistered, poisoned by calomel, and a
hundred other vile drugs which were never designed
by God for the human system at all, than to use that
pure element which is of all others incomparably the
best, and which was designed for man's universal use.

Debility may be much prevented by frequent ablutions in tepid, cool, or cold water, according to the
patient's strength.   If a person is far gone with consumption, I would certainly not use the coldest water ;
I would, however, in all cases, use it somewhat cool.
It is most surprising to witness to what an extent the
patient's strength may be supported in this way.
Pursuing this plan, many are brought to believe that
they are certain to obtain a cure, so great is the benefit experienced.   After having been very weak, and
quite confined to the house, they became able to walk
miles, and bear it well ; and this improvement may
continue for months.   Still, however, it must be acknowledged that, in many cases, the patient must, in
the end, sink ; yet it is a great comfort to keep him
as well as may be ; and if life is desirable at all,
under such circumstances—and the instinct of natur
teaches us the duty of fighting disease to the ve
last—it is a great satisfaction to keep him able to l
about in the open air as long as possible.

"One thing of which I am convinced," says Dr. Billing, of London, the very able author of a work entitled "First Principles of Medicine," "is, that the true principle of treating consumption is to support the patient's strength to the utmost. I am satisfied," says this author, "that the want of exercise induces a languor which makes consumptive patients wear out faster than if permitted to ride or walk, according to their strength, in the open air."

Dr. Billing further observes, that "some years ago, a gentleman, of the name of Stewart, adopted the rational mode of treatment, with which he had considerable success; but because he could not work miracles, his plan was unjustly depreciated. His method was entirely tonic, and especially the cautious use of cold and tepid ablutions of the skin, a modification of cold bathing—a remedy which is found so uniformly beneficial in promoting the resolution (cure) of scrofulous tumors."

Dr. Elliotson also strongly recommends bathing in this disease. "I saw a young gentleman," he observes, "whose brother died of phthisis. He expectorated blood at the same time as his brother; and they appeared equally disposed to the disease. In one it run on very fast, and he died. The survivor was spitting blood continually, and the pupil of his eye was large. I prevailed upon him to begin the use of the shower-bath, and he has done so all the winter. The result is that he has lost his cough, spits no more blood, and is now a strong young man. No doubt, if he take care of himself, and commit no excess of any description, he will go on well. I do not know of any means so powerful, in hardening the body, as the cold shower-bath."

There is no magic, I will remark, as to the particular form of bathing. Any good ablution—the dripping-sheet, as it is called in our hydropathic works, the affusion of water, the washing of the body in a wash-tub, or merely by wet towels and the wet hand—all of these are good modes. The shower-bath, it is to be remarked, is one of the most severe of all; hence great care should be exercised in its use.

Preventing debility, then, we find to be the most effectual mode of treatment, in pulmonary consumption; and for this object bathing, in connection with proper exercise, is the most effectual known means.

CHAPTER XXI.

Treatment of consumption continued.—Sea-voyages.—Their advantages and disadvantages.—Erroneous notions concerning the effect of moisture in consumption and other diseases.—Consumptive patients generally improve at sea, notwithstanding the great amount of moisture in sea air.—A tendency to pulmonary hæmorrhage appears to constitute no objection to sea-voyages.—Testimony of Sir James Clark.—Experience of Dr. Andrew Combe as to the effects of sailing, in consumption.—Some of his opinions controverted.—Sea-sickness.—Its phenomena and effects.—It cannot of itself be supposed to cause any good.—Those who go to sea should select as large and well-ventilated a ship as possible.—Good effects of sailing much owing to the perpetual exercise to which one is subjected.—Long-continued voyages the best.—Sea-sickness does not generally occur in bad cases of consumption.—Sailors are not much subject to this disease.—Atmospheric changes.—The milder seasons the best for most consumptives.—A change is of itself often beneficial.

Sea-voyages in consumption.—Concerning the advantages and disadvantages of sea-voyages in consumption, there have been differences of opinion among writers on this disease. A sea-voyage, in the temperate and warmer latitudes, has certainly many advantages, as well also as disadvantages, when compared with journeying, or remaining on land. The disadvantages are length of time that the patient is necessarily confined to the close, impure, and debilitating atmosphere of the sleeping places, the want of good vegetables and fruits, and fresh food generally; a longing for the society of friends; and a too great sameness in the daily circumstances. But all of these evils, it is held by many, are more than compensated by the favorable circumstances which attend a trip at sea.

Moisture has been often regarded as being especially pernicious in all consumptive cases, and doubtless many physicians, who have sent consumptive patients to sea, with the expectation of their being benefited, have not been aware of the fact that, on every part of the ocean, even in the driest seasons, the atmosphere is exceedingly humid. Heavy dews fall almost before the sun sets. Moisture penetrates almost every thing, even to the innermost parts of the ship's lading. Musical instruments, such as the violin, violincello, guitar, etc., which have resisted the air well on shore, become so permeated by moisture, that they swell, and are not unfrequently rent asunder thereby. Fruits and vegetables, also, decay very soon ; and that all this happens in consequence of the moisture, and not from the effects of sea air, as some might suppose, is proved by the fact that sea air is exceedingly pure, and pure air is the same every where, either on the mid-ocean, on the highest mountain-tops, or in the valleys.

Notwithstanding the great amount of humidity to which seafaring consumptive patients are exposed, we find that they generally grow better, and this, notwithstanding the unfavorable circumstances of the seafaring life. Colds, too, are very seldom taken at sea ; and it is notorious among seamen that, if a person has a bad cold on land, just before sailing, he is likely very soon to get rid of it, after going to sea.

It is proper, however, to remark, in this connection, that the changes of *temperature* on the ocean are generally much less sudden than on land. The climate is always more equable at sea than in the same latitudes on shore.

A tendency to hæmorrhage from the lungs would be reckoned, by some, as forming an objection to a sea-voyage. Reasoning beforehand, it might be supposed that the retching and vomiting to which the seafaring are often exposed, would have a tendency to bring on the difficulty in question. But such is not the fact, and it may, I think, be set down as a safe rule of practice, that going to sea is one of the best possible means that can be resorted to in this state of the system. Any thing that will improve the general health—and going to sea generally accomplishes this object—will aid in preventing the hæmorrhagic tendency alluded to. Dr. Clark tells us that Dr. Peebles of Edinburgh, Scotland, whose long residence at Leghorn gave him a favorable opportunity of observing the effects of sea-voyages on consumptive patients sent from England to Pisa, met with many examples where hæmorrhage had existed. And this, Dr. Clark tells us, was also the case in most of the examples which came under his own observation. The circumstance of the patient being subject to pulmonary hæmorrhage, in the early stages of the disease more especially. is not, therefore, to be considered as affording any objections to a sea-voyage.

Sailing, and riding on horseback, the two remedies which have, perhaps, the oldest and most general repution in treatment of consumption, Dr. Combe regards

9

as owing much of their influence to their exciting the cutaneous function, and equalizing the circulation. He tells us that he himself " became ill in the month of January, 1820, and soon presented many of the symptoms of pulmonary consumption. In spite of the best advice, he continued losing ground till the month of July, when he went by sea to London, on his way to the south of France ; but, finding himself unable for the journey, he was obliged to return from London, also by sea. Being extremely liable to sea-sickness, he was squeamish or sick during the whole of both voyages, so much so as to be in a state of gentle perspiration for a great part of the time. After this he became sensible, for the first time, of a slight improvement in his health and strength, and of a diminution of febrile excitement. Some weeks afterward, he embarked for the Mediterranean, and encountered a succession of storms for the first four weeks, two of which were spent, in the month of November, in the Bay of Biscay, in a very heavy sea. For more than three weeks he was generally very sick, and always in a state of nausea ; and during the whole time, although his head was repeatedly partially wetted by salt water, and the weather cold, the flow of blood toward the skin was so powerful as to keep it generally warm, always moist, and often wet with perspiration, forced out by retching and nausea. The result was, that on entering the Mediterranean at the end of the month, and there meeting fine weather, he found himself, though still more reduced in flesh, and very weak, in every other respect decidedly improved ; and on his arrival in Italy, at the end of seven weeks, recovery fairly commenced, after about ten months' illness; and, by great care, it went on with little interruption till the summer of 1821, when he returned home."

I do not, however, agree, in all respects, with Dr. Combe, in his explanation of the good effects of sea-sickness in consumption. Sea-sickness is one of the most horrible and unnatural feelings to which the human body is ever subject. I do not believe that it does any good to pass long weeks, and even months, as is sometimes the case, with all the horrors of this malady. It cannot certainly do one any good to be almost constantly disturbed in sleep, and to pass many nights in succession, either almost without any repose, or with the most unrefreshing sleep imaginable. The utter horribleness of sea-sickness cannot be conceived of only by those who have experienced it. I cannot, therefore, believe that all this retching and vomiting, soreness of the abdominal muscles, headache, and unutterable depression of the spirits, can cause any good whatever; but, on the contrary. I believe that the prolonged fasting, in connection with the constant exercise caused by the motion of the ship, which persons are thus compelled to undergo, is the true source of the great benefit which is often derived at the time of being sea-sick.

Persons who go to sea for consumption, as indeed from any object whatever, cannot be too careful in selecting as airy a ship as possible, and the best ventilated rooms. Most of the sleeping places in sailing-vessels, even in this day of improvements, are horrible places in which to spend the long and often dreary nights at sea. I have envied even the second-cabin passengers, who were sometimes put in rooms poorly enough furnished, where their windows were left open a greater part of the time. Comparing this with the close and unventilated state-room, furnished no matter how expensively, the occupants of the former have been in a paradise compared with the latter.

A great source of the benefit to be derived from a sea-voyage, doubtless, is the perpetual muscular exercise to which one is subjected in a ship at sea. We are constantly in motion. We can neither walk, stand, sit, or even lie down in our berths, without being subject to much muscular motion. The importance of this source of benefit, has, I think, been often overlooked.

I am informed by intelligent sea-captains, that long voyages, as to the East Indies and to China and back, do much more good than simply going to Great Britain or France. The time, they say, is too short in which to effect any considerable good in confirmed cases of pulmonary disease ; and that it is only by a long voyage that any great and permanent good is to be expected.

It is to be remarked, however, that although most, if not all, consumptive persons who go to sea, appear, for the time to be benefited, the relief is often only temporary. Many persons with this disease do not become sea-sick at all, and if sea-sickness be an advantage, which it doubtless is, because of the fasting which it compels persons to undergo, if for no other reason, many must lose the advantages that would otherwise thus be-gained. I think it will be found, that in bad cases of consumption, as also bad cases in diseases of whatever kind, sea-sickness rarely, if ever occurs. If this is known to be correct, we may regard sea-sickness as a sort of test whether a consumptive invalid may be materially benefited or not. It is plainly true, I think, the most unhealthy persons are, as a rule, the least liable to be affected by sea-sickness. I would admit, however, that the diet and general regimen of the individual have much to do in causing sea-sickness.

Sailors not often subject to the disease—Sailors appear very seldom to have consumption. I admit that they are not a long-lived people, and many of their habits are sufficiently bad to account for these circumstances, but their comparative freedom from consumption is a remarkable fact. This I attribute in part to their springing from parents of hardy constitutions, and such as have from necessity lived upon simple fare and in simple habits of life. But their immunity from this disease is still more to be attributed to their constant exercise, more especially with the arms and chest, thereby bringing the lungs into active play. This too, it is to be remarked, is carried on wholly in the open air.

Atmospheric changes.—Sudden changes of weather, from warm to cold and damp, appear always to affect consumptive invalids unfavorably. We find often that persons who can get along very well during the milder months of the year, experience great difficulty as the season of sudden changes approaches. A more equable temperature of the ocean, doubtless contributes in a high degree to the advantages of voyaging. Persons experiencing much difficulty of respiration when on land or at the seaside, will often be very

sensibly relieved by sailing only so far from the shore
as to be beyond the immediate influences of the land
breezes.   The temperature at sea when beyond sound-
ings, is in a great measure regulated by the mass of
water, the range of temperature of which is very
limited.   Hence there is an exemption from the influence of those sudden and great vicissitudes of heat
and cold so common to our own climate, and which
appear to be extremely prejudicial, in all descriptions
of pulmonary disease.

Consumptive invalids coming from the country to
the city of New York appear for the time generally
to be benefited by the change.   Indeed, I have seen
no exceptions to the rule; and I presume the same
would be true of all large cities which are surrounded
by a country of such changeable climate as that of
New York.   The air of the city in the cool and colder
months—and it is this season to which I refer—is
milder and more equable by night and by day than
the country about.   The inhabitants are shielded from
the winds by the buildings, and the many fires serve
in some measure to moderate the atmosphere.   I have
known persons who were in the habit of coming down
the Hudson river from Albany frequently during each
year, who could always bear well with the city air,
but on going to Brooklyn heights, where the atmosphere is remarkably fresh and bracing, the cough to
which they were predisposed was certain to grow
worse; and so manifest were these symptoms, they
have refrained from remaining over-night in Brooklyn, although they had relatives residing there who
had a right to their company.   This refers, it will be

understood, to the cool and cold seasons of the year only.

I would not be understood, however, as recommending, as a general thing, a residence in the city either for consumptive or any other cases. I regard all large cities as being the great ulcerous, plague spots of the earth; so unhealthy, indeed, that were not their population constantly fed by an influx of new-comers from the country, they would in time literally die out of disease. There is more consumption too, we have every reason to believe, in cities than in the country. But all this does not militate against the fact which I have mentioned in regard to the transient amelioration of consumptive symptoms by persons passing, in the cool and cold seasons, from the latter to the former.

A change from one latitude to another appears of itself often to be sufficient to cause a mitigation in the symptoms of this disease. This, indeed, appears to be true in some cases where the change is from a good to a bad atmosphere—from a healthy to an unhealthy location. And this apparent improvement—which can be reckoned upon only for a short time—must be owing in great part to the effects upon the mind. The more a person thinks of his cough, the more it is likely to continue; and on the contrary, when he goes among new scenes and new objects, his mind being taken fron himself, the cough abates.

CHAPTER XXII.

Treatment of consumption continued.—Effects of climate and fresh air.—Consumption far more common in Great Britain and the United States than in Russia.—Winter residences in relation to this disease.—Patients should be careful of going away from the comforts of home.—Persons in this disease catch at every thing which promises the least hope.—The greater sensitiveness of the body to cold when extensive ulceration exists.—Cold both a tonic and a debilitant, according to circumstances.—It is, however, as a general thing, a tonic.—Moderate warmth appears to agree with a very feeble consumptive patient best.—In very advanced states of this disease life may doubtless be prolonged by going to a warmer climate.—Personal observations of Sir James Clark.—Great mortality of consumption in Bristol, England.—Different localities compared. —Relative mortality of consumption in the larger cities of the United States.—Different estimates of authors.—Few, comparatively, who wish to change their locality have sufficient pecuniary means to enable them to do so.—Most persons must, therefore, do the best they can at home.

ALL authorities agree that consumption is incomparably more common in Great Britain and in the United States than in the more severe climate of Russia. "The lungs suffer rarely among the Russians," says Sir James Clark, "except in public schools, and among those who adopt the European dress and fashions."

I have already observed that a change from one latitude, or from one place to another, is, of itself, often beneficial in the disease we are now considering. But that there is much error in the world in regard to the influence of air in consumption, is, I think, very evident. A brief consideration of this important subject will now be entered into.

Winter residences.—It appears to be a prevalent idea, both with the people and the profession, that going from colder climates to warmer, during the winter season, is beneficial in consumption; and facts seem to warrant this conclusion. But 'n advanced stages of the disease, when tubercular disease of the lungs has become fully established, it must be admitted, humiliating to the profession though it may be, that no real benefit is to be expected from a change of climate, or indeed from any circumstance in which the individual may be placed. It should be a serious question with every consumptive person, who proposes going away from the comforts of home, on a long journey, among strangers, whether he may not receive more harm than good. Not even money is capable of buying those attentions which a sick man often needs; and for this reason, doubtless, many a one has been injured, rather than benefited, by changing his residence to a warmer climate, which, under more favorable circumstances, would have been of some benefit, and in some cases might prove effectual. Let, then, those who are far gone with this dreadful disease, resolve upon remaining under the watchful care of friends, and amid the comforts of home.

It is, I am aware, peculiarly characteristic of this disease, that patients cling to every thing which seems to afford the slightest ray of hope. Indeed, it is often, perhaps generally, very difficult, until almost the very

9*

last moment of life, to convince a really consumptive person that he is in any danger from the delusive disease. Well may it be said of this affection, " a dying man catches at a straw." "The medical adviser," says Dr. Clark, "when he reflects upon the accidents to which such a patient is liable, should surely hesitate, ere he condemns him to the additional evil of expatriation; and his motives for hesitation will be increased, when he considers how often the unfortunate patient sinks under the disease before the place of destination is reached; or at best arrived there in a worse condition than when he lived in his own country, and doomed shortly to add another name to the long and melancholy list of his countrymen, who have sought, with pain and suffering, a distant country, only to find in it a grave."

It will be found a rule, I think, to which there can be few exceptions, that where extensive ulceration has taken place in the system, and from whatever cause, there is a much greater sensitiveness to cold. If this observation be correct, it is an important consideration, in each individual case, whether or not the ulcerative process has actually commenced. If it has not, and yet there is a great predisposition to it, the winter of the Canadas, northern United States, and Great Britain, would doubtless, in many instances, be better than a warmer climate. Cold, it should be remembered, is a tonic to the living system—a permanent tonic; unlike medical tonics, which by use become unavoidably, in the end, debilitants. True, cold may be so severe as to debilitate; but this is the abuse, and not the use of the remedy. In accordance

with this, we find in at least some cases, where a strong predisposition to pulmonary consumption exists, and where many of the symptoms are already present, persons are benefited by being more exposed to cold air.

On the other hand, where ulceration has already commenced, and especially in it have gone to a considerable extent, a warm, genial, sunny climate appears to agree best with the invalid. A comfortable temperature is doubtless the best, as well as the most agreeable, where the pathological condition of which I am speaking exists.

In certain cases, which are not too far advanced, life may doubtless be preserved, for many years, by a constant residence in a mild climate, and by carefully avoiding, at the same time, all imprudence in diet and general regimen, and by adopting that course of hygienic management throughout, which is best calculated to preserve the blood in a mild and uninflammatory state. Dr. Clark tells us that, during his residence abroad, he met with several invalids laboring under this chronic form of disease, who passed their winters in Italy, with infinitely more comfort and enjoyment of life than in England. And I myself have had a number of patients, who have had, to say the least, a strong predisposition to consumption evidently existing, who assure me that when they have left our northern country, to go to such parts as the Gulf of Mexico, some portions of Florida, the Carolinas, and Virginia, they have got through the winter better and more comfortably in every respect than could have been done at the north. But I apprehend that, after all, the imagination has a good deal to do with many of these cases; and besides, human beings are not willing to go to a considerable expense without wishing to believe that they have beeu. compensated therefor.

I am not sufficiently acquainted with this subject to give an opinion as to what locality is best calculated for winter residence for the consumptive; but this much I may safely affirm, that the location, wherevei it be selected, should be of dry, sandy soil, with pure soft water for drink. Such locations, I am told, are to be found at different points on the Gulf of Mexico, between Mobile and New Orleans, and also in various parts of Mississippi. An idea that some have advanced, namely, that aguish districts form a good residence for the consumptive, is erroneous. Always, the purer the air and the better the water—that is, the purer and softer—the better the locality, not only for the consumptive, but all other individuals, provided the temperature be such as to do no violence to the system. In regard to purity of water, it may be observed that, in the region of Bristol, England, one of the mildest and best, as far as the temperature is concerned, the water is exceedingly bad; and here, as I have elsewhere observed, there is greater mortality from consumption, and that too among native inhabitants, than of any other locality of which we have a record.

The climate which Dr. Clark considers of all others the best suited to consumptive patients generally, is that of Madeira. According to meteorological observations, comparing the climate of this island with that of the more favorable situations on the continent of Europe, it appears that the winter temperature is considerably higher and more equable, and the summer heat much more moderate, than at any of these places. Consequently Madeira has this advantage over many other places—that the patients may reside there during the whole year, which would be an object, in many cases, for a residence. But a single winter in any locality, however favorable, cannot be expected to bring about any very great benefit. The two places, which, from the character of their climate, approach most nearly to Madeira, are, according to Dr. Clark, Teneriffe and the Azores. The climate of the latter, in particular, is said to be remarkably mild and equable. That of Bermudas is changeable, and holds out more disadvantage to the consumptive invalid. "The summer climate of the whole shores and islands of the Mediterranean," this author remarks, "is unsuited to consumptive invalids, and indeed is known by experience to be so pernicious to them, that sailors and soldiers attacked with the disease in the Mediterranean fleet, and garrisons of Malta, etc., are sent to England on the approach of summer."

As regards the number of deaths in the four largest cities of the United States—New York, Philadelphia, Baltimore, and Boston, the average annual proportion of the general mortality was, according to the estimate of Dr. Emerson, of Philadelphia, made a few years since, as follows: New York, one in 39.36; in Philadelphia, one in 47.86; in Boston, one in 44.93; in Baltimore, one in 39.17; and that the average of the mortality from consumption alone, to the general mortality, was, in New York, one in 5.23; in Philadelphia, one in 6.38; in Boston, one in 5.54; in Bal-

timore, one in 6.21. According to Dr. Hayward, of
Boston, the deaths from consumption, in proportion
to the whole number, as shown by an estimate made
for ten years, from 1831 to 1841 inclusive, the deaths
in Boston, from consumption, were one in 7.587; in
Philadelphia, one in 7.482; and in New York, one in
5.952. Thus, it appears, authorities differ somewhat
in their estimates, and, indeed when we compare all
statistical writers that have made estimates in relation to these cities, it is very difficult to ascertain
which is most subject to consumption. It is evident,
however, that Boston is by no means so unfavorable a locality as many have supposed. We may, indeed, I think, safely conclude that the chance is as
good in that city as either of the others mentioned.
Dr. Chapman, of Philadelphia, who is regarded as
high authority, considers the native population of that
city as being nearly exempt from this disease. "Comparing Philadelphia with New York, Newport, and
Boston," he remarks, "equally remote from the sea
and the mountains, it comparatively escapes the austere winds of the one, and the cold blasts of the other,
maintaining a more regular and moderate temperature
than the latitude of its position would seem to warrant.
That our bills of mortality exhibit a number of deaths
from this disease, cannot be denied, but most of these are
negroes and foreigners—and it must also be known that
all chronic pectoral affections are reported, with little
discrimination, under the title of consumption. It is at
least a fact," continues Dr. Chapman, "that in the
whole circle of my acquaintance, wide and intimate
as it is, there is hardly a native family who has the

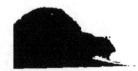

consumptive taint, or who for years has lost a member by this disease." But, on the other hand, Dr. Dunglison, who is equally good authority, says, " that such, certainly, has not been the result of his experience, except in the Philadelphia Hospital, where, for obvious reasons, the proportion of foreigners is large." In private practice, the great number of consumptive cases that have fallen under his notice, has occurred among the "native population." Moreover, the negroes—who fall victims to it in great numbers—are natives, in as large a proportion, perhaps, as the whites who inhabit Philadelphia.

It should, however, be remarked, as an important consideration in reference to consumptive individuals changing their locality, that there are few, comparatively, who can avail themselves of whatever advantages might thus be gained. Even in our northern United States, the population of which is, on the whole, far more independent in pecuniary matters than that of any other country on the face of the globe, very few indeed have the means that would enable them to journey for months a long way from home. It becomes, then, a serious consideration with the majority of consumptive invalids as to what they can best do, under the circumstances, at their own homes.

CHAPTER XXIII.

Treatment of consumption continued.—Exercise.—Valuable remarks
of Dr. Parish.—General effects of exercise on body and mind.—It
should be made a pleasure instead of a task.—It is best when per
formed in the open air, and not alone.—Exercise should be moder
ate when taken immediately after a meal.—The different modes of
exercise.—Walking.—Walking over mountains.—Advantages of
this practice.—It should be graduated according to the strength.—
Riding on horseback.—This was in great repute anciently.—Sydenham and Dr. Lambe.—It is one of the best possible modes.—
Riding in carriages.—Swinging.—The good effect of this doubtful.
—Dancing.—The use of dumb-bells.—Shuttlecock.—Graces.—
Spinning wool.—Farming, gardening, woodsawing, chopping, and
the more useful forms of exercise generally best.—Exercise of children.—Remarks of Dr. Clark.

In the North American Medical and Surgical Journal (1830), there is an article by Dr. Parish, from
which the following is an extract, the doctrines of
which are far in advance of the profession generally,
even at the present time.   The extract is as follows:

"Vigorous exercise, and a free exposure to the air,
are by far the most efficient remedies in pulmonary
consumption.   It is not, however, that kind of exercise
usually prescribed for invalids—an occasional walk or
ride in pleasant weather, with strict confinement in
the intervals—from which much good is to be expected.   Daily and long-continued riding on horseback, or
in carriages over rough roads, is, perhaps, the best
mode of exercise; but where this cannot be com-
manded, unremitting exertion of almost any kind in

the open air, amounting even to labor, will be found highly beneficial. Nor should the weather be scrupulously studied. Though I would not advise a consumptive patient to expose himself recklessly to the severest inclemencies of the weather, I would nevertheless warn him against allowing the dread of taking cold to confine him on every occasion when the temperature may be low, or skies overcast.

"I may be told that the patient is often too feeble to bear exertion; but, except in the last stage, where every remedy must prove unavailing, I believe there are few who cannot use exercise without doors; and it sometimes happens that they who are exceedingly debilitated find, upon making the trial, that their strength is increased by the effort, and that the more they exert themselves, the better able they are to support the exertion."

We read in the sacred volume that it is necessary for man "to eat bread in the sweat of his brow." By this we are to understand that physical exercise is implied. How beautiful is this provision of nature; that the very means which we are to put forth for acquiring an honest maintenance on the earth, is also calculated to promote both healthfulness of body and peace and happiness and contentment of mind. This is a lesson which a selfish, diseased, and suffering humanity has yet to learn.

"Were I to mention the remedy," says Dr. Sweetser, "which promised most in the onset of consumption, I should say, daily, gentle, and protracted exercise in a mild and equable atmosphere. * * * Though exercise in the open air," continues this able writer

"may not be expected to cure confirmed phthisis, yet,
if judiciously pursued from day to day, the strength
will hold out better, the individual will be rendered
more comfortable, will retain more sources of enjoyment, and his existence will probably be longer
protracted than it would have been under confinement."

Exercise, to cause its best effects should not be performed solitarily. Man is a social being. We read
of its having been said, "It is not good for man to
be alone." The mind during exercise should be as
much as possible pleasantly engaged. Exercise to do
its greatest good must be made a pleasure instead of
a task. Those who are interested in botany, mine-
ralogy, and other branches of natural sciences, and
have the means and leisure at their command, cannot fail of finding pleasant objects of pursuit. Journeying through pleasant portions of the country, or to
foreign countries, where "sight-seeing" can be enjoyed to the fullest extent, has a most excellent influence
on those who have strength, and can avail themselves
of such advantages. Would that all poor patients—
a class too, which forms the great majority of cases—
could have these blessings.

To cause its best effects, exercise should be moderately and continuously as the patient can bear. Too
much and too violent exercise is certain to debilitate
the consumptive patient, and so does inevitable harm.
Persons are far too apt to do too much one day, and
then remain idle the next. Moderate and habitual
exercise should be the rule.

As to the best times for exercise, the early part of

the day, when the system is most vigorous, and after the sun has risen high enough to dispel the cold and damps of evening, is to be regarded as on the whole the best. At sea, we need not fear so much from dampness, but on land the temperature between day and night varies much more. For this reason, it is necessary for consumptives to be careful of night air on land. Exposure to the hot sun in the hot weather should also be avoided.

If exercise be taken immediately after eating, it should be of a very mild kind. Gentle exercise always promotes digestion. It must be remembered, too, that what may be moderate exercise for one, may be far too great and fatiguing for another. Each should carefully judge for himself, and the exercise should always be graduated according to the habits and powers of the individual, and to his present condition of health.

Of the different *forms* and *modes* of physical exercise, it is proper that something should be said, and I must here remark, that the tendency with many appears to be the seeking of that which is complex, and not easily understood, rather than the simple and natural modes. People are too apt to confide in dumb-bells, gymnastic academies, ten-pin alleys, and the like —things good enough in their proper place—to the neglect of walking in the open air, tilling the ground, woodsawing spinning, weaving, washing, bread-making, and things of a similar nature. Honest labor with the body is not at all *genteel* at the present day. " The sluggard will not plough by reason of the cold ; he shall, therefore, beg in harvest and have nothing."

This principle holds as good in regard to bodily health as elsewhere.

Walking.—This is said to be the most independent means of exercise, and it is certainly one of the best. Walking is pre-eminently a natural means of locomotion. It brings a large number of muscles into play, and at the same time, when practiced out of doors, as is usually the case, gives us the additional advantage of fresh air and light. These, as I have elsewhere said, are very important agencies in the restoration and preservation of health. Walking shakes off sleep in the morning; it increases the appetite, and aids digestion; it gives vigor and elasticity to the body, and cheerfulness and contentment to the mind.

Walking over mountains, for those who are able to endure such an exercise, is one of the best possible means of giving strength to the lungs, and the system generally. The air is pure, and in consequence of the exertion required, a large amount is necessarily inhaled. Long journeys, performed on foot, have, also, been found most valuable to consumptive patients, who are not too far gone in the disease. Dr. Combe remarks, " I was myself sensible of advantage from this kind of exercise during a Highland excursion. The necessity of frequent and deep inspirations, and the stimulus thus given to the general pulmonary circulation, had an obvious effect in increasing the capacity of the lungs, and the power of bearing exertion without fatigue. Even when I was wearied, the fatigue went off much sooner than after a walk of equal length on a level road, and was unattended with the languor which generally accompanied the latter. In

fact, the most agreeable feeling which I experienced during the whole time was while resting after undergoing, in the ascent of a hill, a degree of exertion sufficient to accelerate the breathing, and bring out a considerable quantity of perspiration. A lightness and activity of mind, and freedom about the chest, which I never felt to the same extent at any other time, followed such excursions, and made the fatigue comparatively light."

Walking, like all other modes of exercise, should be timed and regulated carefully in accordance with the patient's strength. It is no doubt true, that many, both among the sick and the well, avoid this exercise as much as they can, more from want of moral energy and will, than from lack of bodily power. Still, it must be admitted that walking may be overdone ; the consumptive may, by doing too much, aggravate all of the unfavorable symptoms in his case. Good judgment and common sense, joined to experience, are the best guides in this matter.

Riding on horseback.—Sydenham, one of the earlier English physicians, looked upon horseback exercise as a particularly efficacious remedy in pulmonary complaints. In reference to the treatment of cough and consumption, he observes : " But the best remedy hitherto discovered in this case, is riding sufficiently long journeys on horseback, provided this exercise be long continued ; observing that the middle-aged must persist in it much longer than children or young persons. For, in reality, the Peruvian bark is not more certainly curative of an intermittent fever, than riding is of a consumption at this time of life." And elsewhere he says : " But the principal assistant in the cure of this disease, is riding on horseback every day ; insomuch that whoever has recourse to this exercise, in order to his cure, need not be tied down to observe any rules in point of diet, nor be debarred any kind of solid or liquid aliment, as the cure depends wholly upon exercise."

The older physicians, however, drew no very nice distinctions between simple coughs—which may arise from various ailments other than pulmonary—and consumption itself. Hence we must make some allowance in their estimate of this exercise. Still, it is an invaluable means, and should, when at all practicable, be resorted to by the consumptive.

This method has a number of advantages over walking ; it can be persevered in longer at a time, without fatigue, to those who are accustomed to it ; it gives a more general or successive exercise to the body, and at the same time it does not over-tax the lungs ; the patient has a more rapid passage through the air, and is for a longer time exposed to its influence, in connection, also, with that of light.

Dr. Andrew Combe relates his experience of the good effects of horseback riding, in connection with other means. He says : " To carry on what was so well begun (namely, by a sea-voyage to the Mediterranean), riding on horseback in the country was resorted to, and that exercise was found to excite the skin so beneficially as to keep it always pleasantly warm, and generally bedewed with moisture, even to the extremities of the toes ; and in proportion to this effect was the advantage derived from it in relieving the chest, increasing the strength, and improving the appetite. A second winter was spent in the south with equal benefit; and in the summer of 1822, riding was resumed at home, and the health continued to improve. The excitement given to the skin by riding was sufficient to keep the feet warm, and to prevent even considerable changes of temperature from being felt, and rain was not more regarded, although special attention was of course paid to taking off damp or wet clothes the moment the ride was at an end. Strength increased so much under this plan, combined with sponging, friction, and other means, that it was persevered in through the very severe winter of 1822–3, with the best effects. For nine years thereafter the health continued good, under the usual exposure of professional life; but in 1831 it again gave way, and pulmonary symptoms of a suspicious character once more made their appearance. The same system was pursued, and the same results have again followed the invigoration of the cutaneous functions, and of the general health, by a sea-voyage, horseback exercise, and the regular use of the bath. These have proved beneficial in proportion to their influence in keeping up warmth and moisture of the surface and extremities."

Dr. Combe, it will be remembered, finally sank with consumption in the year 1848, and although his disease could not be considered as ever wholly cured, still the benefit he derived from the means he so judiciously adopted, well rewarded him for the efforts put forth. And had his health not been thus improved, he could, in all probability, never have written those able and invaluable works which he afterward did.

Riding in carriages.—When the lungs are weak, and the individual has not the strength to enable him to walk with advantage, riding in a carriage may often be rendered a beneficial exercise. "It calls into more equal play all the muscles of the body, and, at the same time, engages the mind in the management of the animal, and exhilarates by the free contact of the air and more rapid change of scene. Even at a walking pace, a gentle but universal and constant action of the muscles is required to preserve the seat, and adapt the rider's position to the movements of the horse; and this kind of muscular action is extremely favorable to the proper and equal circulation of the blood through the extreme vessels, and to the prevention of its undue accumulation in the central organs. The gentleness of the action admits of its being kept up without accelerating respiration, and enables a delicate person to reap the combined advantages of the open air and proper exercise, for a much longer period than would otherwise be possible."

Swinging.—This, as an exercise in consumption, has had a certain degree of reputation with some. It is, in some respects, like sailing. I consider this of doubtful benefit. It is apt, I think, to injure the brain.

Dancing has been reckoned on, by some, as a means of invigorating the muscular system. It is not, however, often resorted to as a mere means of exercise. It is generally practiced too long at a time, and not often enough, to be productive of any considerable good. Waiving the question of morality, I do not consider this mode of exercise nearly as good as many others. It has the disadvantage of being performed within doors, generally in close and confined air, and at late hours of the night. The rooms, too, are almost necessarily dusty—a circumstance which must always operate, to a certain extent, against the well-being of the lungs. Practiced in the daytime, out of doors, as is common in France, dancing may certainly be made an invigorating exercise.

Dumb-bells, when not too heavy, and not too violently used, are serviceable, as an in-door exercise, for strengthening the arms and chest. Persons generally practice this exercise too violently, and not long enough at a time. Dumb-bells " do harm occasionally from their weight, being disproportioned to the weak frames which use them ; in which case they pull down the shoulders, by mere dint of dragging." In resorting to this, as in all other in-door exercises, the windows and doors should always, when practicable, be thrown open.

Shuttlecock is an exercise that calls into play the muscles of the chest, trunk, and arms more especially, and is therefore good for those predisposed to consumption. If females will persevere, and learn to play with the left hand, as well as with the right, they will find it an excellent mode of preventing spinal curvature, and thus of invigorating not only the whole spinal column, but the system generally.

The play of *graces* is similar to that of shuttlecock, and is also well adapted for expanding the chest, and giving tone and vigor more especially to the upper parts of the system. Both of these exercises are very useful, if practiced in the open air.

Spinning wool, at the common hand-wheel, is one

10

of the best possible exercises for females. It not only gives free movement to all the muscles of the arms, chest, and trunk, but amounts also to a large share of exercise of the whole body.

Chopping and sawing wood, are, for those who are sufficiently strong to endure such exercises, invaluable means of warding off consumption. It must be admitted that exercise, which is performed merely *for exercise*, is never so satisfying to the mind as that which is of itself intrinsically useful. All modes which are resorted to merely as exercise, become soon tedious to the mind, and individuals are not willing to pursue them. Tilling the soil, gardening, fruit-raising, and most of the forms of manual industry, are far preferable, as a general fact, to the more artificial modes of exercise. I would not, however, lose sight of the fact, that man is by nature a social being, and needs at times recreation of the body, as well as of the mind.

Exercise of children.—As a means of preventing scrofula and consumption in children, Dr. Clark gives us the following excellent advice : " When the child has acquired sufficient strength to take active exercise, he can scarcely be too much in the open air ; the more he is accustomed to it, the more capable will he be of bearing the vicissitudes of the climate. If children are allowed to amuse themselves at pleasure, they will generally take that kind and degree of exercise which is best calculated to promote the growth and development of the body. When they are too feeble to take sufficient exercise on foot, riding on a donkey or pony forms the best substitute ; this kind of exercise is at all times of infinite service to delicate

children ; it amuses the mind, and exercises the muscles of the whole body, and in so gentle a manner as
to induce little fatigue. Young girls should be allowed and even encouraged to take the same kinds
of exercise as boys ; it is chiefly the unrestrained freedom of active play that renders them so much less
subject to curvatures of the spine and other deformi-
ties than girls—a large proportion of whom are more
or less misshapen, in consequence of the unnatural
restraint which is imposed upon them by their dress
and imperfect exercise."

CHAPTER XXIV

The treatment of consumption continued.—Inhalation.—Meaning of
the term.—Facts and principles on which the practice of inhalation
is founded.—Advantages of this method.—Ill effects of confinement
within doors.—When and to what extent is inhalation available?—
Method of performing it.—Instruments, and directions for their
use.—Playing on wind instruments as means of inhalation.—Public
speaking and reading.—Their advantages in preventing pulmonary
disease.

By "inhalation" is meant a method of exercising the
chest and lungs, through means of drawing in a more
than usual quantity of air, which is again expelled
slowly and with an effort of the muscles concerned
in the respiratory function.   Thus, if we take a common goose-quill, each end of the hollow part of which
is cut off so that it forms a tube, and hold this, with
some degree of compression, in the mouth, and breathe
through it, either inwardly or outwardly, or both, we
in a measure, and in proportion as we exert ourselves,
give an artificial exercise to the chest and lungs.
This principle has, in different ways, been taken
advantage of by practitioners of the healing art, to
give tone, vigor, and greater volume to the parts of
the living body concerned in the respiratory process.
   The facts on which this mode of practice is based,
are the following: It is a matter of observation that
those classes of persons who are, by their occupation

or modes of life, compelled most to exert these muscles and parts about the chest—such persons, for in
stance, as the various out-door workers noticed in the
tables of M. Benoiston, concerning the Parisian hospitals, in another part of this work—are the most free
from consumption. Singers, and public speakers, too,
by reason of their exercise, often gain great power
and volume of the chest and lungs. Men, also, who
play much on wind instruments, tell us that, instead
of being weak-chested, as when they commenced,
they have grown vigorous and strong under the exercise, the general health, at the same time, becoming
much improved.

In accordance with these physiological facts and
principles, inhalation has been instituted.

"An extraordinary, but most undeserved reputation," says Dr. Ramadge, "is bestowed on various
substances, mechanically received into the lungs, in
a state of vapor. Among these I may mention
tar, iodine, chlorine, hemlock, turpentine, and many
other articles of a stimulating or sedative nature. I
attach little or no importance to any of them. If
benefit is derived, it is, in almost every instance, in
consequence of some such effects as the following .
pulmonary expansion, to a degree sufficient to exert
an influence in bringing into contact the surfaces of
those early cavities which are most invariably formed
in the summit of the lungs ; pulmonary catarrh, or its
common consequence, as vesicular emphysema (infla-
tion), in both of which the lungs acquire an unusual
magnitude ; in the latter more especially." This quotation gives an explanation of the benefits that are to be

derived, *mechanically*, from the method which we are now considering.

But there is another advantage gained by inhalation, and a very important one in the cure of consumption. The air breathed may well be compared to food in the living body. Food gives us blood, but air is necessary in order to make that blood pure. Air may be said to be food to the blood. If the lungs breathe but little air, the blood must of necessity be but poorly purified. If that air be impure also, the blood, evidently, cannot be so perfectly formed. The good condition of the blood depends much, therefore, upon the *quantity* and *quality* of the air we breathe.

If an individual be confined in a close and badly ventilated room, so that his lungs become enfeebled by want of the proper stimulus of pure air and exercise, we find that soon the whole frame becomes weak. There are, it is true, a variety of causes concerned in bringing about this result; but one of the most efficient among them all is the lack of good air for the daily and constant purification of the blood in the lungs.

When, and to what extent is inhalation available? If extensive cavities have already been formed in the pulmonary tissue, we cannot, unfortunately, in the great majority of cases, look for any permanent improvement, whatever may be the means employed. Still, in these unfavorable cases, surprising relief will often be afforded by inhalation in connection with other suitable treatment, and life may in many instances be thus materially prolonged. Such persons should begin the practice with caution, since whatever tends to over-exercise the lungs under such circumstances will only tend to hasten on more rapidly the fatal work. Players on wind instruments, singers, and public speakers have often brought on fatal hæmorrhage from the lungs by an excessive effort in these exercises. But any individual may, if he will but observe carefully, be enabled to go on safely in this matter. If inhalation over-fatigues the system, or if it excites much coughing and expectoration, or any other unpleasant symptoms, let him desist for a time ; at least, let the efforts be made milder. Thus by beginning carefully, doing each succeeding day a little more than on the preceding, a great deal of good may be accomplished in most cases.

Inhalation performed two or three times daily, and half an hour or an hour at each time, has been found in a few weeks to work a wonderful change for the better in the chest. " Externally, the muscles concerned in respiration become manifestly enlarged," says Dr. Ramadge, " and the bony compages of the chest, both before and laterally, visibly increased ; while at the same time, the natural respiratory murmur will be heard internally far more distinct than ever. Such has been the increase of size which the chest, in young persons especially, has undergone through the exercise of inhalation, that I have known individuals, after inhaling little more than a month, require their waistcoats to be let out. It is a fact incredible to one who has never been at the pains to measure the chest, or examine its shape," continues this author, " what an enlargement it acquires by the simple action of breathing for the time above stated (a half hour

two or three times daily) backward and forward
through a narrow tube of a few feet in length." It is
said that on measurement of the chest, its circumfer-
ence may be increased within the first month of inhaling to the extent of a whole inch.

Means by which inhalation is accomplished.—A
method which has been adopted by some in inhalation,
and one which has been particularly recommended by
Dr. Ramadge, of London, is to make use of a tube of
rather small calibre, several feet in length. The patient
breathes both inward and outward through this apparatus, and in so doing necessarily gives exercise to all
the parts concerned in respiration. Another method
is to have a small tube of silver, wood, or some other
material, with a calibre of from an eighth to a six-
teenth of an inch, and about three inches in length. At
the outer extremity of this tube a valve is arranged so
as to allow the free passage of air inward to the lungs,
but which partially closes as the air is expelled. Thus
the lungs are kept inflated a longer time than would
ordinarily be the case in the act of expiration. This,
then, amounts to an artificial exercise of the parts,
and resembles very nearly the action of the respiratory organs of an individual playing on a wind instrument. I do not however see any particular advantage in the tube containing a valve over the simple
form or even a common goose-quill. We need exercise in drawing *in* air as well as in forcing it *out*.

These breathing tubes have been sold at a very
great price, compared with their cost. If a practitioner holds forth that he will give advice *gratis*, but
must sell twenty-five or fifty dollars' worth of appara-

tus and drugs before he can do any thing, it does not look very well, certainly, as to point of honesty. It would be a better mode—and one too which would succeed better in the end—if he should sell his articles at a fair valuation, and at the same time have pay for his professional services direct. But there are all manner of means by which dishonest men cheat the community, and in no one thing is this carried on more effectually, or more successfully, than in matters of treating the sick.

I have myself designed a form of breathing tube which I consider much more convenient, and better fitted to the purpose intended, than any I have yet seen. It is made of silver, and will be furnished at a price not to exceed $1 50. At the same time I must tell my readers that I consider a common goose-quill, with its ends cut off, quite as good as any other tube. But if the *silver* is an object, and if an individual considers that he will persevere more with the use of that which is costly, he can easily obtain tubes at from $1 50 to $5 00, as he may choose. On the other hand, if he prefers to go upon Poor Richard's plan, that "a penny saved is as good as two earned," he may carry in his pocket the common goose-quill, and if he will but persevere, may succeed just as well as with the more costly apparatus.

In conclusion, on the subject of the breathing tube, I would remark, that patients should not reckon too much on its advantages. Nor should they neglect bodily exercise, or any of the other well-known means of regaining lost health. Above all, they should not use it to excess. It should be looked upon as *one* of

10*

the various means by which life may be prolonged and rendered more comfortable—a means which has an abuse as well as use.

Playing on wind instruments.—Those who are predisposed to weakness of the chest and lungs, will do well, if they will but commence in season, to select some wind instrument of music to practice on, as a means of invigorating the parts mentioned. The flute is one of the best of musical instruments, and is, moreover, one that is easy to learn. As a general thing, however, those instruments which require the mouth to be closed in the act of blowing them, are best. The clarionet, the bugle, and French horn are instruments of this class. When the blowing is performed with the mouth closed, as is the case in the use of those instruments, the lungs are more inflated, and the exercise greater, than in the use of the flute. But it should be particularly remembered, that these exercises may be misused; persons have been killed by them—that is, by practicing too violently, by doing too much at a time, or by adopting them at a time when the lungs were too weak to bear the exertion. A little care, and the exercise of good common sense, however, will generally be sufficient guides in all such exercises.

Public speaking and reading aloud.—It is said that the celebrated CUVIER was in the habit of ascribing his own exemption from consumption to this practice. At the time of his appointment to a professorship, it was believed that he must necessarily fall a victim to this disease. The habitual exercise of lecturing gradually strengthened his lungs, and improved his general health so much, that he was never after threatened with any serious pulmonary disease. Mr. O. S. Fowler, the able and well-known lecturer on Phrenology, tells us that there is no doubt but that, if he had not commenced speaking in public, and giving phrenological examinations in private, he would long ago have died of consumption. " I find," he remarks, " its habitual practice, if not indispensable in order to arrest the progress of this consumptive tendency, at least highly beneficial to health, and a powerful strengthener of the lungs." A medical lecturer of London gives us the following testimony : " We know ourselves, from personal experience, that often, when preparing to go to a lecture, a languor has crept upon us, inducing an unwillingness to exert ourselves. We have gone—the lecture has commenced—the mind was called into action—a perspiration broke forth on the brow—the circulation was equalized—and, at the conclusion of the lecture, the languor was gone." Hence, also, this writer recommends " reading to one's family in the evening, as an excellent practice, and one tending much to sweeten social life."

Public speaking may, however, like every other good exercise, be carried to excess. Clergymen, who are often in the habit of speaking two or three times on a Sunday, and then little or none at all during the week, and who, at the same time, use but little physical exercise of any kind, are often injured by it. Sore throat, bronchitis, weak chest and lungs, and even consumption itself, are thus sometimes evidently brought on.

CHAPTER XXV.

The treatment of consumption continued.—The processes of water cure.—Water drinking.—Importance of water as an agent of life.—Effects of water taken internally, in fevers and other inflammatory diseases.—Rules to be observed.—The injection, or clyster.—Modes of using it.—The abreibung, or rubbing wet-sheet.—Its mildness and general applicability as a form of bath.—The towel-bath.—The sponge-bath.—The shower-bath.—Rules for its use.—General directions concerning baths.—Bath by affusion.—The plunge-bath.—How often should we bathe?—The half-bath.—The head-bath.—The nasal bath.—The mouth or oral bath.—The lein-tuch, or wet-sheet.—Mode of applying it.—Wet compresses, bandages, and fomentations.—The cooling, the warming or stimulating, and the soothing wet compresses.—Their use in pains of the chest.

THE processes of what is popularly termed the "water-cure," being eminently valuable as a means, both of prevention and cure of consumption, according to the nature of the case in which they are applied, I have deemed it advisable, in this work, to enter somewhat into detail concerning them. And I here re-affirm what I have elsewhere inculcated, that this treatment, which includes, in its detail, water, air, exercise, diet, and clothing, is the best of all known methods in this most formidable malady of which I am writing. Those who desire to peruse a more detailed account of these processes, are referred to the "Water-Cure Manual," written by the author of this volume.

Drinking of water.—The human body, as a whole, by weight, consists of about 80 parts in the 100, of water. Even its drier portions, as bone, muscle, cartilage, ligament, and nerve, contain a large proportion of this fluid. The blood has about 90 parts in the 100, and the brain nearly the same proportion. Without the presence of water in the living body, food would not become digested in the stomach; no chyme would be elaborated, to supply the chyle, or chyle to form the blood. Respiration, circulation, secretion, nutrition, perspiration, elimination, neither of these could take place in the human system without the presence of a large proportion of water.

The living body may be compared to a perpetual furnace, which has a tendency, constantly, by evaporation, to become dry. If food and water are, in every form, withheld, the individual grows parched and feverish. In a few days, delirium supervenes, and, in about three weeks, he dies. But if water be taken according to the demands of thirst, no fever or delirium ensues, and life goes on more than twice as long as when both food and drink are withheld.* These facts

---

* In the "Transactions of the Albany Institute," for 1830, Dr. McNaughton relates the case of a man, named Reuben Kelsey, who lived on water alone for fifty-three days. "For the first six weeks, he walked out every day, and sometimes spent a great part of the day in the woods. His walk was steady and firm; and his friends even remarked, that his step had an unusual elasticity. He shaved himself, until about a week before his death. and was able to sit up in bed till the last day." Kelsey was twenty-seven years of age at the time of his death, and, during his fasting, evidently under the influence of delusion. At the beginning of his course, he assigned as his reason for so doing, that he would be furnished with an appetite when it was the will of the Almighty he should eat.

Barn-yard fowls, kept from food and drink, do not survive the ninth day. If water is allowed them, they reach the twentieth day.

show us, most conclusively, the great value of water as a drink.

It is not, however, proper to speak of water as a nutriment. True, it is immediately concerned in most or all of the transformations constantly going on in the system ; but that water is ever decomposed, or chemically changed, in the living animal, has not been proved ; nor have we reason to believe that such is ever the case.

Water, besides being the best of all drinks, is, as an internal remedy, the greatest of all medicinal substances. We can scarcely give a lecture, enter a neighborhood, or even a family, and introduce the subject of water, but that we are at once told of remarkable instances of cure, which the narrator has known to take place, through the drinking of water. The patient was very sick ; learned physicians declared, " For his life, he must not touch cold water." Every thing fails ; the man grows worse—is given up ; and, in the long, dark night, to give some small relief from his raging thirst, water is administered. The friends tremble for his safety ; but he appears to grow better, and more is given. Sleep and perspiration ensue. The patient lives—" *in spite of cold water,*" shall any one say ? Or, perhaps, in his delirium, he has broken over all bonds, and quaffed, suddenly and deep, of the fluid which, above all earthly things, he craved ; or, by stealth, hire, or threat, he accomplishes his object. Who ever knew a patient in high,

These experiments can be easily tried ; but, as the principle is well established, no possible good would result ; and none but the most heartless barbarian would repeat them.

burning fever (not induced by over-exertion) killed by cold water? Many have been saved; but more, alas! incomparably more, have been lost for the want of its use.

These facts all go to show the importance of water, both as a curative and prophylactic agent, in pulmonary consumption. Only pure soft water is to be used. By this means, the cough and feverishness may be often modified, to a truly wonderful extent.

Rules for drinking water.—A very good rule for the healthy, and such as have active exercise, is to drink, except in fatigue and exhaustion, as thirst demands. Patients may have the general direction to take at such times, as when the stomach is empty, as much as can be conveniently borne, which will generally be from six to twelve half-pint tumblers in the whole day. Feeble persons must not go on very rapidly at first. If they have been accustomed, a long time, to hot drinks, they should, on commencing, make small beginnings, gradually training the stomach in the new way. Wonders may thus be accomplished, if the patient can have system and perseverance enough to proceed.

The better statement for invalids, perhaps, is, "exercise as much as may be without causing too great fatigue; by this means, the system becomes invigorated and warmed; more fluid is thrown off, more is needed, and more relished; so exercise and drink as much as you conveniently can."

Patients in the later stages of consumption will always find themselves much the better if they will omit the supper, and take only pure soft water instead

By this means *the* cough and feverishness may be often modified to a truly wonderful extent.

The injection, or clyster.—This very important part of the water-treatment is as old as the healing art itself, but in the endless complications of the remedial means of modern times, almost any irritating or disgusting fluid, other than pure water, is preferred. A variety of instruments for administering injections are now manufactured, varying in price from four to five dollars. The cheaper kinds, if well made and used with some degree of dexterity, answer a good purpose. Every person should have access to one; no lady's toilet is complete without it. Contrary to the common notion, a person, by the exercise of a little skill, can easily use this remedy without assistance. It is in no wise painful, but decidedly agreeable, and affords, in a variety of complaints, speedy and efficient relief. Thousands suffer incalculably from constipation, year after year, when the use of this simple means would give the greatest relief, and thousands more are in the daily and constant habit of swallowing cathartic and aperient drugs, Brandreth's pills, castor oil, magnesia, blue pill, mercury, and so through the long chapter, that irritate and poison the delicate coats of the stomach, and exert their pernicious influence throughout the numberless lanes and alleys of the system, destroying the healthy tone of the tissues, deranging the nerves, and thus causing a state of things incomparably worse than the disease itself, and rendering even that more and more persistent.

Most persons may and should use this remedy cold. A beginning may be made with the water slightly warmed. In obstinate cases, lukewarm water effects the object quicker and with greater certainty than cold. It may be repeated again and again, in as great quantity as is desired. Some prefer the clyster before breakfast; others immediately after; the former, I believe, on the whole, to be the best. A good mode, too, is to take a small injection, a tumbler full, more or less, that is retained permanently without a movement before morning. This is very soothing to the nervous system, aids in procuring sound sleep, and by its absorption, in the coats of the bowels, dilutes acrid matters therein, tonifying and strengthening likewise those parts, and aiding materially in bringing about natural movements; but invaluable and efficient as is this remedy, let no one persist in those habits of diet, such as tea and coffee drinking, the use of heating and stimulating condiments, greasy and concentrated forms of food, etc., that tend so certainly to constipation and irregularity of the bowels.

In all forms of looseness of the bowels, as diarrhœa, dysentery, cholera morbus, cholera infantum, and the like, this remedy is most excellent. In many a sudden attack, injections, sufficiently persevered in, will suffice quickly to correct the attack, and this when, in the ordinary treatment, a course of powerful drugging would be deemed indispensable, that would result perhaps in death. This statement will cause sneering, I know, but it is no fancy sketch. The thoroughly washing out, so to say, the lower bowels; by which also the peristaltic or downward action of the whole alimentary canal is promoted, and by the absorption or transudation of water, its contents are moistened and diluted, and the whole of the abdominal circulation completely suffused, by that blandest and most soothing of all fluids, pure water. I say all this is sufficient to effect, in all such cases, a great amount of good ; and whoever understands well the sympathies and tendencies of these parts of the human system, will at once perceive the truth of that I affirm. So, also, in constipation and obstructions of the bowels, when no powerful cathartics that any one dare venture to exhibit, can be made to act, this simple remedy is effectual in bringing about the desirable object.

In any of these cases, if there is debility, and especially if it be great, whether the patient be young or old, the water should be used of a moderate temperature—not above that of the blood (98° F.), nor very much below that point. Even if there is high inflammation and much heat in the bowels, water at 90 or 95°, persevered in, will readily bring down the temperature of the parts to a natural state, as may be determined by placing the hand upon the abdomen. The patient's feelings of comfort as to warmth or cold are a good guide. With these precautions as to temperature, etc., the injections may be repeated for an hour, or even hours upon the stretch.

The abreibung, or rubbing wet-sheet.—This is one of the mildest and most convenient forms of a bath. A large linen sheet, of coarse material, is wrung out in cold water, and, while dripping, one or more assistants immediately aid in rubbing over the whole surface. This is continued, briskly, three, five, or more minutes, until the skin becomes reddened, and the surface in a glow. The system is then made dry with towels, or a dry sheet. Frictions with the dry hand are also very useful. If the patient is feverish, much friction is not required—the sheet is repeated often.

In determination of blood to the head, the lower extremities being generally cold, the rubbing-sheet tends to restore an equilibrium of the circulation. The rubbing wet-sheet, in principle, is easily administered to patients in such a state of health as to render it necessary for them to remain in bed. The person lays upon a blanket that may be afterward removed; a portion of the system is rubbed, first with wet towels, followed with the dry. This part is then covered, and the other extremities disposed of in the same way. The water should be moderated according to the strength of the patient. All who are able to walk about, to insure warmth, should take the water cold.

If a person is very much fatigued, and covered with perspiration, he must be careful how he meddles with the cold bath. But if the fatigue has not gone too far, although there is perspiration, the rubbing wet-sheet is one of the most soothing, and, at the same time, invigorating modes that can possibly be found. Such as have become exhausted from public speaking, strong mental efforts, watchings, and the like, are greatly benefited by the rubbing wet-sheet. If at any time the surface is cool, dry frictions or exercise are to be practiced, to induce warmth, before it is used. If a person from debility fails of becoming warm, he is well wrapped in dry blankets a half hour or more, and when sufficiently comfortable the rubbing sheet is again given, to promote the strength. Frictions, with the dry, warm hands of assistants, are always good in these cases, to help to insure warmth. If a person finds himself remaining cold in the lein-tuch, he should omit that, until the use of the abrei-bung, exercises, etc., enables him to get warm. The tonic effect of the rubbing-sheet is most serviceable in night perspiration and debilitating sweats.

The towel-bath.——By means of wet towels we may take almost any where a good bath. With a single quart of water we can do this, even in a room carpeted ever so nice, without spilling a single drop. The towel-bath may seem a small matter; but we find none, but the most lazy, who, once accustomed, are willing to relinquish its use. Small matters oft repeated and long continued accomplish much. A *little* medicine is taken day by day, and, at length, health fails, and death is the result. Tea, coffee, tobacco, wine, etc., are used in very *small* quantities, and the teeth become dark, and decay; the head aches, the hand trembles, and the spirits fail. So good influences, however small, in the end accomplish great results.

Sponge-bath.——Some like to stand in a tub, and use a large sponge out of which the water is pressed, and made to pass upon the head, neck, and shoulders, and other parts. We may pour water from a cup, basin, or pitcher, if we choose. There appears no particular advantage in the sponges — the water is what we need.

The shower-bath.——This is often wrongly used. As physicians are becoming generally more impressed with the importance of water, they not unfrequently say to a patient, "Take the shower-bath." The patient, a lady, perhaps, is very weak. Medicine enough to make her so, quite likely has been given, and a good bill run up. Last of all, the order comes, " Take the shower-bath ;" about as philosophic a prescription as to say to a person in severe constipation, and not at all acquainted with the doses of medicine, " Take Croton oil." Of this most powerful of all purgatives, every one would, of course, take too much. Within a few years, since baths are getting to be the fashion, I have known a number of persons materially injured in consequence of this loose kind of advice. A great many patients are too weak to take the cold shower-bath. Milder means must be used.

The shower-bath should never be taken upon the head. Some can bear it ; but, in all cases, it is better to wash the part. The head should never be beaten by water, or any thing else. Most men have an idea that taking it upon the head is necessary, to prevent rushing of blood to the part. Cooling the head is, of course, good for this, and, if the bath has but little force, the head is, in many instances, benefited. But it may be beneficially acted upon indirectly, as by the foot-bath, which is excellent to relieve headache. The hip-bath is easily managed, so as to cause the same effect. So, also, the shower-bath, upon any or all parts of the body, but the head, may be made to cause the same result. Now the blood at the feet is cooled, and now it has arrived at the head. The blood is rapidly coursing through the system ; and thus, by cooling it, we very soon affect the most distant part.

If the person has strength enough, and does not

take the shower-bath upon the head, he will find no difficulty in its use. It is a very valuable and convenient mode ; and many persons have, by this simple means, been most wonderfully restored. And yet some water-practitioners are so prejudiced, that, if a patient commences telling them the benefit he has derived from its use, they at once fall into a rage. It is easy, in these cases, to see where the shoe pinches: they have committed themselves beforehand, and been talking of what they know but little about. If I have, myself, taken some hundreds of the shower-bath, and prescribed it to hundreds of others (as I have), I ought to know more concerning its effects than those who have seldom or never attempted its use. I do not say that a shower-bath is the best that can be ; but I contend, that, properly managed, it is a most excellent mode. The pouring of water, or the small stream, of the same quantity and force of the shower, I hold is, in most cases, the best. I go, as I always have done, for *avoiding* the shock, although this is generally advocated as being the principal good of the bath. The pouring, and the small stream, much less than the shower, produce this result.

General directions concerning baths.—Persons who are under the necessity of commencing the use of water, without the advice of a physician (and most persons in chronic disease, with the most perfect safety, may), should begin very cautiously. It is so easy, at any time, to increase, that there is no need of hurry in the matter. " Haste makes waste." Begin by merely washing the surface once, daily. If you are very weak and sensitive, use the water at

70° F., or even 80°, and, if it is at 90°, it is yet cooling—cold water, in effect, and very mild in degree. It is easy, then, to lower the temperature, day by day, as you find you can bear. Rub the skin thoroughly, to excite activity in this part. The warmer it becomes, and the better the circulation, the more grateful is water, and the better the effect accomplished. Very soon one can commence taking the shower, small stream, or douche, upon a part. Take it, first, upon a single limb, or two, next upon all the limbs, then upon a part of the body, and, finally, upon the whole, except the head. In this way, any one, who is able to walk about, may gradually and safely accustom himself to the shower, or small douche bath. Most persons are apt to wish to proceed too rapidly, and, in so doing, fail of bringing about the best results. If disease has been a long time accumulating, as is almost always true, time must be given for nature to do her work. We may aid her in her efforts, but to force her is impossible. Many invalids, of course, have strength to proceed much more rapidly than I have indicated for those who are very weak. But, I repeat, those who practice upon themselves should proceed cautiously and, as it were, feel their way.

If one bath per day is found useful, soon a second may be ventured upon, and, finally, a third, or even a fourth. Weak persons go fishing voyages, and, in many cases, soon become able to remain much in the water, the whole day, and half of the night. If a crisis appears, we may know nature is doing her work. The treatment must then be moderated according to the degree of the critical action present.

Bath by affusion.—A person may stand in a wash-tub or any convenient place, and by means of a pitcher, cup, or hand-basin, pour water upon the neck and shoulders, and thus take a very excellent bath. This simple way will indeed be found, as a general thing, better than the portable shower-baths. These are very apt to get out of order, although some of them are very good.

Fifty years ago, Dr. Currie, of England, performed wonders by the affusion of cold and tepid water, graduated in temperature according to the strength of the constitution. In all the varieties of fever he adopted the mode; so in small-pox, measles, scarletina, as well as in convulsive diseases and in insanity. It is now acknowledged by the highest authority in that country, that Dr. Currie's mode was attended with greater success than any other previously known.

Plunge-bath.—In sea, river, and lake, as well as by artificial means, bathing and general ablutions have been practiced from time immemorial; as a matter of luxury, religious observance, purification, prevention, and cure of disease, bathing has been resorted to in every period of the world. So efficacious has this simple means proved in the healing of the sick, that not a little superstition has been mingled with it. Springs and wells have often been supposed to possess some mysterious power, and have, therefore, been named after some patron saint. The world has loved mystery and marvelousness, has ever been wandering from simplicity and truth.

How often should we bathe?—There appears to be as good reason for the daily cleansing of the whole

surface as of the hands and face. I have before written, every sick person, in whatever condition, or however weak, should have the whole body rubbed over, with wet cloths, sponges, etc., at least once each day. In some cases, great caution will be required, in order that the bath be performed safely. Let those who have lain for days upon a sick bed, without any ablution, as is usually the case in the ordinary modes of medical practice, try, when the body is warm, the rubbing it, part by part, over the whole surface, following, briskly, with dry cloths, and then covering it warmly, according to the feelings of comfort, and they will find it a most effectual tonic, as well as an application productive of the greatest comfort. Physicians, generally, have yet many simple lessons of this kind to learn.

Let every individual, then, old and young, male and female, sick or well, have a daily bath ; and, in case of indisposition, of whatever kind, let there be more, instead of less attention, given to this practice.

The half-bath.—This may be used as one of the mildest of water processes, or as one of the most powerful. An ordinary bathing-tub is a very good apparatus for the purpose. A good-sized washing-tub will answer very well, if there is nothing else at hand. The water is generally quite shallow in this bath— from three to six inches. Priessnitz's half-baths are made of wood, four to five feet long, about two and a half feet wide, and twenty inches deep. This simple contrivance is one of his most powerful means—that by which some of his highest triumphs are achieved. The water is generally used of moderate temperature,

11

as 60° to 70° F., and when long continued, is changed, as it becomes warm from the heat of the body.

Head-bath.—From time immemorial, cooling and other applications to the head have been much depended upon in that violent and dangerous disease, phrenitis, or inflammation of the brain. When all other means had failed, certain obstinate affections of the head have been known to give way by a constant stream, or affusion of cold water, upon the part. In headaches, convulsions, delirium tremens, the delirium of fever; in epilepsy, rheumatism of the head, diseases of the eyes, ear-ache, deafness, loss of smell and taste; and in epistaxis, or nose-bleed, this highly energetic remedy is brought to bear.

In taking the head-bath, the person lies at length upon a rug or mattress, with perhaps a pillow under the shoulders. A broad, shallow basin, or bowl of some kind, is used. The back and sides of the head are, in succession, placed in the water. It may be taken for five minutes to a half hour, or even more, according to the case. The whole head should be well rubbed and dried, if there is no inflammation to combat.

Those who are under the necessity of going to excess in literary labors, or have much mental effort to put forth, will find great benefit from affusions upon the head, and the head-bath. Not unfrequently a troublesome headache will at once give way, by merely washing with cold water the part in which the pain exists.

The nasal bath.—In catarrh, colds in the head, and

in diseases of the nasal passages, the sniffing of water up the nostrils is to be performed. The water should be drawn back and ejected by the mouth, to obtain the best effects. This is a little disagreeable at first; but one soon becomes accustomed to it.

The mouth, or oral bath.—For inflammation in the gums, mouth, throat, and palate; in slimy secretions from the throat, stomach; in toothache, catarrh, colds, and chronic hoarseness, garglings, and baths for the mouth, are of great service. Pauley, a merchant of Vienna, has been thought singular for his zeal in recommending this bath. Clergymen and others, who suffer hoarseness by much speaking, will find that holding very cold water in the mouth, until it begins to grow warm, and then ejecting it, and by frequently repeating the process, much benefit will be obtained. Falling or elongation of the palate, in which it is now so much of a professional hobby to clip off the part, the gargling sufficiently with cold water will be found a never-failing remedy. Coughs and tightness in the chest may often be essentially relieved by this bath. In mucous secretions from the throat and stomach, by ejecting the water a number of times, it will surprise those who have not witnessed the remedy, to see the amount of slimy secretion thrown off.

The sitz, or hip-bath.—Convenient tubs, wooden or metallic, are constructed for this bath; but an ordinary wash-tub answers very well. The article should be large enough to admit the motion of the arms in rubbing the abdomen, sides, and hips, first with one hand, and then the other. Water enough is used generally to come pretty well up the abdomen. The more movement and friction, while in the bath, the better. It is more convenient if the tub be elevated two or three inches from the floor. Some undress completely, and place a blanket or sheet over the upper part of the body; but oftener the parts only of the person, to be exposed to the water, are uncovered. In a variety of ailments, this bath is highly valuable. It may be made one of the most powerful of all of the hydropathic modes. Like all other powerful applications, it should be made only after digestion is nearly or quite gone through with.

As a tonic to the stomach, liver, bowels, womb, spine, etc , this bath is highly useful. In constipation, and other irregularities, it is famous. Those of sedentary habits will find its use of rare service. It may be taken for five, ten, or more minutes, according to the demands of the case.

The leintuch, or wet-sheet.—The usual mode of applying the wet-sheet is thus: a number of woolen blankets are spread evenly upon a bed or a mattress; a sheet, of cotton or linen material (linen is the more cooling), is spread smoothly upon the blankets; the patient then lays at length upon the sheet. This is lapped over from side to side, and made to cover the whole surface; the blankets, one by one, are, in like manner, adjusted, drawn tightly, and well tucked under each side. Large pins, or tapes, may be used, to secure these coverings. The blankets should be well arranged about the neck and feet, to prevent evaporation and too great chilliness. A down or feather bed is sometimes put over the whole, and tucked under, the more effectually to retain the warmth. If there is a tendency to coldness of the feet, these may be left covered with the blankets only. Faithful rubbing them with the hand, is a good mode. Working and rubbing them one against the other, is serviceable; and, rather than allow these parts to remain a long time cold, as is sometimes done, it would be better to place moderately warm bricks, or, better, bottles of warm water, etc., to them; and the same may be said of any part of the system. Some fear warm applications, in water-cure, seeming to believe that every thing must be of a cold, chilling kind. The fact is, *warm* applications, though seldom needed, are, under certain conditions, as natural, as scientific, as the *cold*, under other conditions. Still, it is always better, as far as possible, to cause the body to create its own warmth.

The wet-sheet is now used, by Priessnitz, only as a cooling means. It may be called a convenient mode of applying a cold bath. His practice is, to allow patients to remain in it only for about twenty minutes at a time.

Some form of bath should be given, after the wet-sheet, not that it is absolutely required in all instances, to be safe, but, on the whole, it is more beneficial so to do. The surface now needs cleansing, and the invigorating effect of cold water. If a person is weak, and not able to sit up, the water should be used tepid, as at 70° or 75° F. Piecemeal, with wet towels, the body is to be rubbed, until dry; and it is better to obtain a comfortable glow. A half-bath may be taken, or a shower, plunge, or spout-bath, as the case may be. As in all other applications, those who have not

the advice of an experienced physician, should begin
with the milder modes, and then proceed gradually
to the stronger, as they ascertain, by experiment, what
they can bear.

Wet compress bandages and fomentations.—These
perform precisely the same office upon a *part* of the
system, as the wet-sheet upon the *whole*.

Cooling wet compresses are such as are changed or
re-wet frequently, until the necessary amount of coolness is obtained. These are applicable to any part.

Warming, or stimulating, wet compresses are, in
their secondary effects, the opposite of the cooling.
Covered, and left upon the part a sufficient length of
time, the surface becomes warm, and even warmer
than is natural, in consequence of the retained heat.
They are therefore said to be *warming*, or *stimulating*.

Soothing wet compresses.—A distinction may be
made between the cooling and the warming. Such
as give no decided sensation of either coolness or
warmth, may be said to be soothing in effect.

Under the head of "pains in the chest," I have elsewhere alluded to the good effects of compresses on the
affected part.

I have thus given a short description of the principal modes of using water, both as a remedial agent
and a preventive of disease. I advise most strongly,
that all who are in any way predisposed to pulmonary
consumption, resort to these processes, according to
the means they have at hand, and the necessities of
the case.

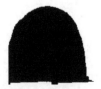

CHAPTER XXVI.

Treatment of consumption.—Case of Miss Lydia Mott, of Albany.—
Mr. Waterman Roberts, of Hartford, Ct.—Mr. Jacob Campbell, of
New York.—Mr. John S. Sunderland, of Penn.—Lyman Sherwood,
of Ia.—Mr. Henry C. Wright, of Philadelphia.

HAVING entered, in the preceding chapter, into an account of the processes of the water-cure, so called, I now propose to give a number of cases in illustration of the effects of this treatment in consumption, and its kindred complaints.

Case of Miss Lydia Mott.—In the Water-Cure Journal of Dec. 15th, 1845, I published the following case of this young lady.

"About the first of October last, my friend, Sidney Howard Gay, of this city, called to confer with me concerning the case of Miss Lydia Mott, of Albany, given up by her physicians, as he was informed, in a hopeless state of consumption. I said to him in substance, as I always do in reference to this disease, that water-treatment is altogether more powerful to save than any other known mode, and that in case a cure is necessarily impossible, the treatment, incomparably more than other, *will prolong life and render the sufferings less.*

"In two or three days after this conversation with Mr. Gay, I received a letter from the sister of Miss Mott, asking my opinion of her case. The sister informed me that the physicians declared her case to be one of tubercular consumption, and that they despaired of medicines reaching her case. She said, furthermore, 'for the week past we have tried the wet-sheet and bandages during the day, with no other result but an apparent suspension of the disease.'

"In one week from this time, I had the pleasure of seeing both the sister and patient at my house in New York. I had advised her to continue the treatment which appeared to be doing so much good, and that as soon as possible, for a change of air, it would be one of the best things she could do to make a journey down to the city. They remained two or three days, Miss Lydia feeling decidedly better from the journey, and having obtained my directions for future treatment, returned home to Albany.

"Concerning the true nature of her disease, there may be some doubt. I am myself not fully satisfied what it was. Up to the time of her commencing water-treatment, she had been under the judicious care of Drs. Ward and Paine, of Albany, and Dr. Bryan, of Troy, as counsel. I have not yet had the satisfaction of conferring with either Dr. Ward or Paine. I met with Dr. Bryan, who told me that when he saw the patient, she had, without any mistake, *hepatization*, as it is called (*hardening*), of the right lung. As to his opinion concerning *ulceration*, I do not recollect. He considered her case a very dangerous one, and he should watch the progress of the disease under the water-treatment with much interest. Drs. Ward and Paine, as I am informed, declared that there was actual ulceration of the lung. Not having seen the patient until she had considerably recovered, I cannot give any positive opinion of my own. There could not have been any mistake as to the *hardening* of the lung; and this alone is dangerous enough without ulceration, which did probably exist. If ulceration did exist, it was caused either by the inflammation and breaking down of tubercles, or it was the result of inflammation of the substance of the lung, causing hardening, and the hardening resulting in ulceration. This, however, seldom takes place, although it sometimes does. The ulceration is by far oftener caused by the inflammation of tubercles, than by inflammation resulting in hepatization or hardening of the part. Whatever was the state of the lung, I am confident there was likewise severe rheumatic pains in the chest, which amounted to a good deal of suffering.

"It is proper here to state more of the history of this case. Miss Mott is a person of very active habits, and during the last spring took a severe cold which settled upon the lungs. This caused a serious illness at the time, and which continued to trouble her very considerably during the whole summer. She did not, as she usually has done, spend a part of the hot season in the country air, but remained actively engaged during the whole of the past hot summer. About the first of September she took again a very severe cold, settling, as before, upon the lungs, and resulting in the dangerous illness described above.

" Beginning now again at the time when she returned home from visiting New York, she continued to use water nearly two weeks longer, at which time I was at Albany, and called according to promise, to

11*

see her. Before commencing at all the use of water, Drs. Ward and Paine very candidly said, that notwithstanding they considered the case now entirely hopeless, they would be glad if water-treatment could be fairly tested, but that themselves, not having given the subject sufficient attention, could take no responsibility in its use. In making this statement, these gentlemen exhibited a degree of candor which we too seldom find. How many physicians are there yet of our country who have at all seen the application of the wet-sheet, and yet very generally they assume to know as much about it as if they had administered it as often as they have doses of calomel. This is not as it should be ; and if they do not choose thoroughly and impartially to investigate the new mode, patients will practice upon themselves, as in such case they should. But to return to the treatment in this case.

"The wet-sheet, as has been said, was used each day. It was wrung from water that was rather mild of temperature, and applied according to the usual mode. It produced a soothing and relieving effect, and was followed by an ablution in water of a moderate temperature. Four well wrung wet towels were arranged about the chest to meet at the side, making two thicknesses of wet linen upon every part of the chest. Over these towels still another moist bandage was placed, and over the whole an abundance of flannels, to retain the warmth. These were worn at first, I believe, only during the day. It would have been still better to have continued them at night also. The effect of the sheet, the ablutions, and the bandages in removing pain, preventing general fever, cough, and night sweats, was indeed wonderful. She improved astonishingly in strength, and, as before said, was able to journey to New York in two weeks.

"During a part of the following two weeks, she is now of the opinion, that she used too much of cold applications; or that, as the general feverishness of the system, and particularly of the chest, was at this time considerably removed, the same applications as before made were not now well borne. The system did not, as before, react sufficiently against the cold. During the most of this second two weeks, the patient thinks she rather lost ground than otherwise.

"In four weeks she came again to the city to remain with us, to undergo a more thorough treatment than could be conveniently carried on at home; besides, she felt that she needed special advice, as new symptoms might arise. The right lung was at this time still very weak. I should have said, that on first seeing her, that is, two weeks from the commencement of water-treatment, the hardening of the right lung had given away considerably, so that the air penetrated some distance downward. At the end of the four weeks there was still much pain through the chest, particularly the right side, and extending to the right shoulder, and under the right shoulder-blade. The right arm could only be used with great difficulty. In the most comfortable situation it could be placed, two or three days were required to a finish a single letter. The treatment by the wet-sheet once daily, and ablutions and bandages, were kept up. In two or three days she was able to bear a mild shower bath, and in two or three days more a small douche. This proved very strengthening, and was powerful in removing pain. At Albany she could scarcely go in the open air at all. The mild air of this city agreed much better, and she was, day by day, able to take more exercise in the open air, and in less than two weeks she could walk at one time some miles without inconvenience, and with benefit. After a few of the first days she took two shower or douche baths daily, besides the one following the wet-sheet, in all three general baths daily.

"After remaining nearly three weeks, she thought, as a matter of experiment, feeling now so much improved, she would make some friends a visit on Long Island. She remained about one week, continuing the daily use of water, and returned still more improved. She could now undergo as much exertion as she had been able to do for years, and has now (Nov. 26th) returned to Albany, after having used water in all about eight weeks, to remain, I hope, in the enjoyment of good health. With the good care she will now observe, there is reason to believe that no recurrence of the disease will take place. Still, it must be remembered, the chest is contracted and weak, and that this will be the part most likely to give way first.

"Food, it should be mentioned, was taken very sparingly. During the first two weeks, it consisted almost entirely of grapes. During the second two weeks, friends had urged that flesh meat should be taken to promote strength; as her health was, if it had been said, to promote pain, inflammation, coughing, expectoration, and weakness, the fact would have been stated. While with us, she partook of farinaceous food, as coarse bread, milk, toast, buckwheat cakes, potatoes, squashes, turnips, stewed fruit, etc., using of animal food only what little was contained in the preparations in which milk was used. No butter, or food in any way prepared with butter, was taken. Salt was almost entirely abstained from. We care not what physiologists tell us from *theory* about the *necessity* of salt. We go for facts. Salt, like other medicines and medicinal stimulants, we choose to abstain from. Miss Mott partook of food but twice a day, and on the whole, the regulation of diet had no small share of effect in her remarkable cure.

" She is now able to endure nearly or quite as much exertion in the open air as she ever has been, and more than most ladies in good health. Time will determine how permanent her cure may be.

" It should have been mentioned that, while upon Long Island, Miss Mott, feeling quite strong, thought she would try the experiment of discontinuing the bandages upon the chest. She found, in less than one day, that she could not yet do without them. A sensation of sinking and weakness in the chest was experienced. It will be best, for a time at least, that the bandages be continued, both night and day, as they have been."

In 1847, I remarked on this case as follows :

" Miss Mott remains yet very well. It should be remembered that, in all these cases of so-called cure of consumption, the lungs remain the weakest part of the system ; and that such persons are, perhaps, of

all others, the most subject to colds. In every chronic
disease of important organs, the best possible cure
that can be effected, yet leaves the part that has been
affected in a condition susceptible to the disease.
This remark applies particularly to diseases of the
lungs; and those who may have the fortune to become cured of such disease, should remember that the
greatest care and perseverance will be required, in
order to enable them to keep tolerably free from colds
and fresh attacks ; and that, in the end, they must, in
all probability, sink with that fearful disease, consumption of the lungs.

" Since making the above remarks on Miss Mott's
case, she writes (March 4th, 1847) : You will be gratified to learn that my health is good, although I still
perceive a little difficulty in my chest. I have not
had any colds this winter. They have been very
prevalent with us."

Up to the present summer (1849), this patient remains well. There is every reason to believe that,
with her very simple and industrious habits, and by
the exercise of good judgment, which she possesses in
an eminent degree, she will yet live to a good old age.

*Case of Mr. Waterman Roberts, of Hartford,
Conn.*—This case of Mr. Roberts was published in
the "Water-Cure Manual," first, in the spring of 1847.
It was given as follows :

"It is due Mr. Roberts to state, that he is only
willing that his name appear in public, because of his
belief that some one, in the condition he has been,
may be similarly benefited as himself. I give Mr.
Roberts' own account :

"I am now forty-five years of age. My habits of life have been decidedly active. My health, until about five years ago, was usually good. My grandparents were long-lived. My father died at the age of forty-seven; my mother at fifty-seven, of consumption. One of my brothers, younger than myself, died a few years ago, at about forty, decidedly of the same disease. My mother had the disease some eight years; my brother about three years.

"Five years ago last November, I was attacked with the lung-fever. For a while before that time, my health had not been as good as usual; but I still kept about. For this attack, I was bled, according to the usual modes in such cases, freely. The bandage became disarranged in the evening of the same day, soon after the bleeding was practiced. I awoke, and found my arm in a puddle of blood, as it were. I immediately undertook to rise from my bed, but fell in the attempt, and fainted. The loss of blood made me exceedingly weak; but I appeared to be, in a measure, free from the fever. However, at the end of about two days, my lung-fever returned with increased violence, and I became delirious. Various means were resorted to; and after some days I began to mend, so as to be about the house a part of the time. I was, however, very weak, and highly susceptible to cold; and could not undertake business until late in the spring. I never again became so strong as before, until after I resorted to the use of water. An obstinate cough followed this attack, and was very bad. I raised, first and last, a good deal of matter, apparently from my lungs. Food, also, disagreed with me; and I lost much flesh. About two years after my attack, I became much reduced, and had frequent night sweats.

"About this time (Feb. 1844), I was advised, by my physician, to take a voyage to the West Indies. I sailed to St. Domingo, and was absent some three months. The voyage appeared to be of benefit, during my absence. My cough was less, the raising less; and I became a little stronger. But, on returning to Hartford, my difficulties soon returned; yet not so formidably, until cold weather again set in. Warm weather appeared then to agree with me best.

"In December of the same year, I became much debilitated and discouraged. By the advice of some of my friends, one in particular, I was led to examine the water system; and, as you will recollect, called upon you for advice. You left it optional with me whether to go home and be treated, or to return to you. The first I concluded to do. I was very thin, and susceptible to cold. You advised me to begin cautiously, with tepid bathing, and a good deal of friction. The wet jacket upon the chest, to be covered with flannel, I was to commence at once. After a few days I was to commence showering with cool water, immediately after the tepid bath. My health was such that I frequently took colds. You recommended that, at such times, I should lay awhile in the dry blankets, to cause warmth, and that I might the better endure the baths. Occasionally, I sweated in the blanket; and perhaps, in a few instances, became weakened thereby.

"For a time, I bathed twice daily. The cool towel-bath at evening acted most beneficially in arresting the night sweats. The wet application worn over the chest night and day, changed three or four times in the twenty-four hours, seemed to allay irritation in the lungs, and to prevent the cough. The effect was very soothing, as well as warming. After some weeks, I at times left off the wet jacket for a day, and was surprised to find that the surface was warmer where the wet cloth had been than elsewhere. Still I felt the need of it for its tonic and soothing effect. You directed me to have no more fire in my sleeping room, and to have it well aired by day. I was also to exercise in the open air daily, and to be out as much as I could possibly bear. It was better for me, you said, to go out even when it was stormy and inclement, than hover over the fire in a hot room. I asked if I had not better take some syrup or medicine for my cough. These I had taken by the quart. You said, ' Nonsense ; the cough will take care of itself, as your strength becomes improved.'

"I was to partake only of plain, coarse food—brown bread especially ; the less meat the better. The coarse bread has been my 'staff of life.' Until I became strong, I used plain flesh meat, and but once a day. I left off tea and coffee, drank only soft water. My appetite had been by turns very poor, but now increased wonderfully. Digestion also improved much. From that time to the present, now two years and two months, I have, with some little drawbacks, been growing firmer in health and strength. For the past eight months, I seem to have been able to accomplish as much, and undergo as great bodily fatigue, as for the same space at any time within the last ten years.

"I feel yet that the lungs are the weakest part; and I sometimes take colds; but I have each time succeeded in throwing them off by renewed treatment, the blanket, baths, wet jackets, injections, etc. The tepid bath, taken usually at from 70 to 75° F., followed by a slight shower, cold, has seemed to be, of all baths, the most beneficial. For the past seven or eight months, I have, as a rule, used the water cold. I have good reaction, and the cooler the air now, the more am I invigorated. Differently from before, I now enjoy the cold weather decidedly the best.

"And now, after having followed the water-treatment for more than two years, although my lungs are not yet free from weakness, and I am liable to serious pullbacks, yet I feel grateful to God, that I have received such wonderful benefit. And I do herein add my testimony, that I have unwavering confidence in the water-cure."

I have heard a number of times from Mr. Roberts, since the above account of his case was published. He has continued, on the whole, very well, so far as I have learned, and I am confident he is still in good health (Nov., 1849); otherwise, I may conclude, I would have heard to the contrary.

Case of Mr. Jacob Campbell, of New York.—Mr. Campbell's case was also published in the Water-Cure Manual, in 1847.

"The case of this gentlemen is certainly, all things considered, a very remarkable one. Mr. Campbell is a resident of this city, engaged (principally at the desk)

at th. bank in the Bowery. He is of very fair, delicate complexion, blue eyes, and auburn hair, a most perfect subject for consumption. The disease is also hereditary in the family, on the father's side. His father's brothers died of it, and he has lost already a brother and sister by consumption.

"Mr. C. is now thirty-one years of age. About one year ago, the present time (15th March, 1847), he called to consult me. He had had a pain, at times severe, in the left lung, for two years. For eighteen months he had raised blood, but not in large quantity. He expectorated a good deal, apparently from the lungs. This exhausted him very much; he was indeed so debilitated that it was with difficulty he could go to and from his place of business, or attend to his labors at the desk. He took colds often, and at the most trifling exposures. He had suffered also a good deal from constipation, and appetite was poor.

" Mr. Campbell could not at the time come to my house, nor could he leave his business. Accordingly, he was under the necessity of doing what he might at home. I directed him to commence bathing, once a day for three or four at first, and then twice per day, with wearing the wet jacket about the chest, to observe strictly the rules of diet, and gradually to go more and more in the open air. There was an immediate amendment in all of his symptoms, and he pursued the regular course for months, continuing business, however, all along. He grew stronger and stronger, and the appetite improved; the wet jacket removed all pain from the chest, the expectoration grew less and less, and the spitting of blood entirely ceased.

Mr. C. now says how he has been as strong all winter as he ever was in his life. Appetite perfectly good for the plainest food, and the bowels regular. The expectoration is not all gone, but he says there is not now more in a whole month than formerly in one day.

"Whether there were actually tubercles that had gone to suppuration or not, it is impossible to say. Mr. C.'s former physician, a man of respectability and experience, declared that tubercles did certainly exist. The result of the treatment has been entirely beyond my most sanguine expectations. It is to be observed, however, that Mr. Campbell persevered in the treatment with a diligence that deserves great credit.

"It seems, then, that this was a case in which the patient fled to the water-treatment, just in time to save life. No one acquainted with that dire disease, could believe that Mr. Campbell would long hold out as things were going. Generally, consumptive patients come to us after all other means have failed, and then it is too late, only they can be invigorated somewhat, and kept incomparably more comfortable (if we may use that term), than by any other known means. There is probably a point at which, if water-treatment were commenced, almost every one could be saved. But after the disease has become deep-seated, we must tell our patients frankly *that in all probability they must sink.*"

Since the foregoing account was published I have often seen or heard from this patient, and he has remained well to the present time (Nov., 1849).

Case of Mr. John S. Sunderland.—The case of this young man, with the accompanying advice, was published in the Water-Cure Journal of Sept., 1848. It is as follows:

"John S. Sunderland, a young man of Newton, Bucks County, Pa., writes us respecting his case the following particulars. He had been much subject to croup when young, and for years had shortness of breath and difficulty of breathing. In the winter of 1845, he took a severe cold, and had also been subject to these attacks previously. He took colds upon colds until 1846, when he had become so weak from constant cough that he was obliged to lie by for some weeks When he exercised or made some exertion, he raised bloody, frothy matter ; the cough was very bad at night. He was subject frequently also to the nose-bleed. In June, 1847, he had an attack of fever. After this left him he had chills two months. For a sore spot in one of the lungs he was ten times blistered by a physician of Philadelphia. He also had a pretty good share of self-dosing in the way of syrups, cough mixtures of the nostrum kinds, etc. Finally, he became so low last winter that he was obliged to keep to the house, and was not able to go up stairs at all. He says he could sleep only in a sitting posture, and often not a half hour in the whole night ; raised much hard phlegm ; appetite sometimes very good, and at others none at all ; had severe turns of nose-bleed, some of which lasted four and five hours at a time. 'I must say I got tired of taking medicine,' he says, 'for on counting up the number of bottles of the different kinds I have taken, I find they exceed fifty, besides the other medicines from the physicians. By chance I heard of water-cure about two months ago. A young man told me that he had received great benefit from the treatment, and he advised me to purchase a copy of your Water-Cure Manual. I immediately obtained one, and thereupon commenced bathing. I was so weak that I could only take a towel-bath at first, and that only with assistance. I regulated my diet according to your directions, and have found great benefit by so doing. I use water as my constant drink; boiled apples and brown bread, pot-cheese, thick sour milk, and boiled rice and potatoes. I have, however, used a little boiled lean meat about once a week. I use no butter or any thing but what is recommended. My appetite, which was before so changeable, has now become so good that I relish well the coarse bread.

"'I have now been two months bathing. Three weeks ago I commenced with the entire bath, in a large wash-tub. With this I make out very well. At first I used the water a little lukewarm, but gradually I have become able to bear it right out of the pump. After bathing, I dress and take a glass of water, and then walk in the open air. I eat my breakfast with an appetite like other people. I can go up stairs now to sleep without coughing, and can rest without being propped up. My cough is a good deal better than it was, but is not entirely gone. I can walk farther than I could for a year. I feel no more trouble of palpitation at the heart, which, before I commenced bathing, troubled me. I have had no trouble of bleeding at the nose since I commenced bathing. I feel

much stronger and better in every respect. I forgot
to mention that I was catching cold at every change
of weather before I commenced the water, but since
that I have scarcely taken any.'

"*Remarks.*—The above case is attested by Thomas
Janney of the above, and further advice is asked for.
Whether the young man can be cured or not is very
doubtful. He has been asthmatic, but there is still
greater trouble in the lungs, as would appear from the
raising of blood and thick phlegm. He ought not to
bathe at all in water as cold as that from the pump.
Let it stand a while in the sun, and use only *soft* water, if it is possible to obtain it. If he continues to
bear it well, he may plunge into water of rain or river-
water temperature once a day, in the morning—not
more. He may take the rubbing wet-sheet (rub *over*
the sheet, not *with* it, as is generally done), forenoons
and afternoons—not oftener. Three or four foot-
baths per day a few minutes each, water not too cold,
and walking after each will be useful. These may be
taken soon after meals, and on going to rest. Washing the neck and chest with the wet hand a number
of times a day, will also be serviceable; but the wet
bandages about these parts few are competent to
manage properly during hot weather. An ingenious
person may use them advantageously mornings and
evenings, but they are almost invariably allowed to
become too warm, and then weakness is the inevitable
result. Persons of this class almost always do too
much with water. They should do little by little, and
keep doing, and especially should they observe the
rules of exercise and diet.

" *Exercise.*—This too is apt to be made too violent. Do little and often, and proceed as you can bear. Horseback riding is probably the best of all forms of exercise for those who have weak lungs. Riding in a carriage is good. Walking also should not be neglected, and if a person has not the means of riding, let him walk and undertake lighter forms of out-door work. Persons have been astonishingly benefited by taking long journeys on foot, going a little way daily, and then increasing the distance as they can bear. Some have been thus cured who could scarcely walk in the commencement of their experiment. The tonic and invigorating effect of the fresh open air, and the light, when not too powerful, is poorly understood. Remember out-door exercise and work constitute the best part of water-treatment, so called, in chronic disease.

" *Diet.*—Our readers already pretty well understand our notions on diet. We hold that the same kinds of food and drink which are best for the vigorous, athletic, and healthy, are best also for the most feeble, only we must graduate the *quantity* according to the patient's amount of exercise and strength. There are all sorts of notions about diet, both in and out of the profession ; that one kind of food is good only for one person, and another kind for another ; in short, that what is one man's meat is another's poison. Is not good brown bread in liberal quantity good for a ploughman ? So if a half pound of it is good for him, a half ounce, less or more, is good for the sickest man if he need nourishment at all. If a teaspoonful, less or more, of Indian or wheat meal water-gruel is good

for a fever patient of a morning, who begins to need nourishment, so is a bowlful good for a ploughman or any other man to go to meeting upon. There is no truth in the old saying, that what is one man's meat is another's poison.

"Any kind, quality, or form of food which is good for one man is good for all men, and under all circumstances, provided they need food at all. Waiving the question of animal food, or rather admitting for the moment its necessity, milk, we contend, is the best form. Sour or loppered is certainly one of the best forms in which it can be used. The German and Dutch people in some parts of this country have seemed to do remarkably well with buttermilk and buttermilk porridge a little sweetened, with other food. All these things, however, must be taken in moderation. Consumptive persons, more than all others, are apt to take too much food. It has been a common saying that nothing disagrees with their stomachs, because they generally feel no trouble in that part. But the mischief, however, is visited in all its intensity upon the poor lungs. So in other diseases, the weakest and diseased parts receive the injury most.

"New milk, as warm and fresh as possible from the cow, has been much recommended by some good judges in this disease. From some experiments in lung diseases we think well of it. But no one should make any great sudden change. Some people who have thought they could not eat milk, find that soon, by help of the water-treatment, they can go at once to great excess, acting as if they thought the more of a good thing they could get down their throats the

12

better. It would seem as if no class of persons thought and reasoned so little for themselves as patients in chronic disease; and no schoolmaster ever had one tenth part of the trouble that the physician of a water establishment has if he takes at all to heart the business in which he is engaged. Consumptive patients, above all others, should be careful in the use of water. If people ever learn to have a tenth part of the confidence in water, air, exercise, and diet, that they have in the ten thousand nostrums that are hawked about by saint and sinner every where, then we may begin to indulge a hope that the great scourge of our country, consumption, will begin to wane away. Now it is on the increase."

I have never heard from this young man since answering his letter.

Case of Mr. Lyman Sherwood.—In the summer of 1848, I received the following letter, from a very worthy relative in the west:

> "HAMILTON, Steuben Co., Ind., *May 12th,* 1848.

"DEAR NEPHEW: I wrote you last summer, and obtained some books on the water-cure, which, I think, have been of so much benefit to myself and family, that I have concluded to write again, and request you to send me the 'Water-Cure for Ladies.'

"When I wrote you last summer, I was impelled by the strongest motives. Your cousin Betsey had been from home, attending the Lagrange Institute; and the young lady with whom she roomed had a brother, about three-and-twenty, between whom and my only child there appeared to be the strongest attachment.

His parents were from New York state—a very respectable family, and members of the Presbyterian church. We could not object to the young man; but we were pained to find his health very poor, with many symptoms of consumption. He had tried apothecary medicine till he became discouraged. He came to our house the first of June, last year, then under the care of a German root-doctor; but his health seemed failing. He had not done a day's work for three months, nor been able, at any one time, to sit up all day. I put your 'Cold-Water Journals' into his hand, and urged him to leave off drinking tea and coffee (he being immoderately fond of the latter), and adopt the use of cold water. When he read of some one getting out of bed and plunging into a cold bath, he said he would not do it for one hundred dollars. I then told him I had, for three months, practiced cold bathing in the morning, and that, instead of killing me, it had nearly cured me of the rheumatism. He returned home, a distance of twenty-five miles; discontinued the use of tea and coffee; and the next morning stripped, and plunged into a creek, near his father's house; rubbed dry with a towel; and returned to the house. His parents were very much alarmed, thinking he would surely kill himself. But, in one week, he was able to commence work moderately. His health continued to improve; and he became anxious to be married.

"Accordingly, your cousin was married to Lyman Sherwood, August 11th, 1847. He then came to our house to reside; and I persuaded him to use the wet bandage to sleep in nights, and in the morning to wash himself in cold water, having no other chance of bathing. His health continued to improve, and his cough to abate; and he gained in flesh remarkably, until February, when there seemed a general disease of the lungs to affect the whole population; and there have been many deaths.

"Since that time, he has been much worse. We have procured a shower-bath. He wears the bandage nights; takes the bath in the morning; and then tries to labor through the day. He has almost constant pain in the stomach; coughs a great deal, and raises much. The matter is not tough, like that of a person with a cold, but seems almost rotten. He has considerable fever nights.

"I am very much afraid he is past help; and yet, if you can form any opinion from what I have written, and think there is any help for him, write us; and if you advise it, he will come at once to your establishment, if he can be persuaded so to do. I do not think he is fully aware of his danger.

"If you can possibly find time to answer this long letter, which you must pardon on account of my anxiety for my son, you will much oblige, etc.

"Yours, with respect,

DELANA BEECHER."

At the time of receiving the above letter, I wrote a somewhat discouraging answer, believing that the young man could not live. I remarked, in my reply: "The case is one which shows well the tonic effects of bathing. We can easily make consumptive persons, who can walk about think they are going to get well; so powerful are the effects of water, when properly used. This young man's life has, no doubt, been prolonged by bathing. He *may* have bathed in water too cold, or too much. But, on the whole, he has been much benefited. Persons with lung diseases should, of all others, be the most careful; and they are perhaps, of all others, must apt to go to extremes. It is singular, too, that they seldom appear aware of their danger until the very last."

Judging from the description of Mr. Sherwood's case, at the time, I did not believe it possible for him to live. I am informed, however, now, in the autumn of 1849, that he has become well; sufficiently so, at least, to enable him to attend to business.

Case of Mr. Henry C. Wright.—This gentlemen, of the city of Philadelphia, went to Graefenberg, in Germany, in the year of 1844. The following account was published by him in a very able and interesting work, entitled "Six Months at Graefenberg," which was issued in London, in 1845. Mr. Wright still remains well in 1849. His account is as follows:

"My lungs, I was assured by my medical advisers, were ulcerated, and my organs of speech and respiration diseased; my chest, which was formerly very full and prominent, had fallen in. My breathing, once deep and strong, was difficult and painful; my sleep, never very sound, much more disturbed than usual. I had a dry and sometimes painful cough for more than a year; a short walk made me perspire, and I was subject to night perspiration. I was conscious of great weakness compared with my former strength; and my constitution, originally exceedingly vigorous, had received a shock from which I never expected to recover. I am forty-six years of age, and such has been the soundness of my constitution and my general health, that I was never confined to the house by sickness one day in my life. I had never been bled or blistered, had never swallowed an emetic or a particle of calomel, nor indeed ten shillings' worth of medicine of any kind. Cold water had been my only drink for fifteen years; no alcoholic liquors, fermented or distilled, no tea, no chocolate, no warm drink of any kind had passed my lips during that time; and I had been exposed to the extremes of heat and cold, from 100° above to 10° below zero (Fahr.), by night and by day, by land and by sea.

But continued public speaking during the last twelve years, in the United States, and in England and Scotland, in connection with Sabbath schools, and for the promotion of teetotalism, anti-slavery, and peace, had at length affected my lungs, and caused a general prostration of my physical nature. For three years past I had worn flannel next my skin in summer and winter, thinking that I could not live without it. I had usually worn cotton, worsted, silk, or fur mufflers round my neck, to keep as far as possible all cold, fresh air from my throat, chest, and lungs. I had used every precaution to keep the pure air from the surface of my body, supposing that health and comfort are promoted by keeping the skin as much as possible from the direct action of the air. As I had for years been accustomed to bathe and wash myself in cold water every morning, both winter and summer, I had no fear of its effects when applied as soon as I left my bed in the morning; yet I was afraid to let the cold air circulate freely about me, not reflecting that if my body could with benefit receive cold water on its surface, cold air could not injure it.

"I commenced the water-cure at Graefenberg, under the direction of Priessnitz, on the 12th of last January. The weather was exceedingly cold, the thermometer (Fahr.) nearly at zero. All my flannels were laid aside; my silk, cotton, worsted, and fur mufflers were thrown off. I was ordered two leintuchs (wet-sheets) daily, one at five in the morning, the other at five in the evening, with a cold bath after each. At first, for about week, I took the abgeshrecktebad (tepid shallow bath) instead of the cold bath, after the leintuch. At eleven A. M., I had a sitz-bath (sitting bath) for fifteen minutes. I wore the umschlag (a damp bandage covered by a dry one) round my body, and changed it four times a day. Every morning before breakfast, be the weather ever so inclement, I walked four, six, or sometimes eight miles, having previously drank six or eight tumblers of cold water. I also took a walk after the sitz-bath and evening leintuch, to excite re-action. This treatment lasted for three months. I afterward took the douche or water-fall bath once a day, and instead of the evening leintuch and cold bath, two abreibungs (wet-sheet baths) at intervals of an hour.

"From the first I found the cure exceedingly stimulating. The various external and internal applications of cold water, the out-door exercise, and pure air, which in my walks I allowed to circulate about my neck, throat, and chest as much as possible, had, during the first three months, a most invigorating effect. A rash appeared upon my neck, chest, and shoulders, and around my body under the umschlag, and was rather annoying from the burning and itching which it occasioned. My cough ceased; I had a voracious appetite; I found that my breathing grew deeper, stronger, and easier, and that I could climb the mountains more rapidly, and with less panting.

"But a painful change was at hand. About the 1st of April all my joints, and especially my knees, began to grow stiff, sore, and weak; walking became painful, and after sitting for a few moments I found it difficult to straighten my knees. I became gloomy and disheartened; but was assured by those about me that these were favorable symptoms, being evidences that the cure was taking effect. The whole surface of my body, even my hands and face, became very sensitive to the touch of cold water. It seemed as if my nerves were laid bare. I had a perfect horror of cold water, a kind of hydrophobia. As the spring advanced, and the weather grew milder but damper, the cure became more intolerable. I found the damp weather of April and May far worse than the cold of January and February. I became afflicted with acute and throbbing pain in my teeth, jaws, and face, for which I was directed to rub the back of my head, and my neck and face with my hands, wet in cold water. I was also ordered to rub my knees frequently in the same way. This was the crisis, and for some weeks I was as miserable as the most enthusiastic admirer of the water-cure could desire. Indeed, I was often congratulated on my misery, which was

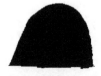

regarded as the prelude to a speedy cure. At the close of April, I had boils on my arms, hands, fingers, and chin, and nearly all over my body. They suppurated and discharged; and during the month of May they all healed, and none have since appeared. I have continued the application of cold water externally and internally, with free exercise in the open air. Since I left off the water as a cure, I take it as a luxury. I feel that all disease is removed from my lungs; my chest has recovered its natural fullness, and my breathing its usual ease and freedom; my cough is entirely gone, and my voice is as strong and deep-toned as ever it was. I think great violence must be done to my lungs before disease can again fasten upon them. What I may yet enjoy of health and physical comfort, I owe, under Providence, to the water-cure, and to the kind friends who, against my will, almost compelled me to go there. During my experience of the cure, nothing surprised me more than the perfect safety with which I cast away my comfortable warm flannels and mufflers. A terrible cold upon my lungs and an increase of cough were the least that I expected; but I was agreeably disappointed. In my walks, for three months, I had no hat or cap on my head, no handkerchief around my neck, not even my shirt collar buttoned. My clothes have often been completely drenched with snow and rain, and my hair filled with snow; but I have not had the slightest cold upon my lungs, nor any which a leintuch or one night's rest has not cured. My only remedy has been to take an abreibung and put on dry clothes on returning to my room to take off my wet clothes. This

12*

simple process has not only saved me from taking cold, but also from the effects of over-exertion.

"After my experience at Graefenberg, I shall never again have any fear of colds, influenza, or fevers, however violent, if I have but the means of applying the water-cure. It is impossible to fear these diseases, after seeing the most malignant fevers so easily and speedily subdued by a remedy that leaves no sting behind. I went to Graefenberg resolved to submit implicitly to Priessnitz's directions. I did so, and was restored to health. I am certain that my long abstinence from all alcoholic and warm drinks, and my disuse of tobacco in all its modes, and of medical drugs, have been powerful aids to my recovery. If any one will make cold water his only beverage, and abstain entirely from the use of medicine, he will find the water-cure sufficient to cure any disease that may assail him, if it be not absolutely incurable, and if he be determined to persevere in whatever process may be requisite for his recovery. But whoever expects to find health by the water-cure while wrapped up in flannels, and lounging on easy chairs and on sofas, in a warm, air-tight room, without personal exertion and activity, will certainly be disappointed; 'or perseverance and exercise in the pure fresh air is an essential element of the cure."

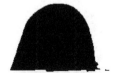

CHAPTER XXVII.

Treatment of consumption concluded.—Animal sensibility as affected by heat and cold.—Interesting facts in relation to the power of habit.—Clothing natural to the human body.—Effects of flannel worn next to the skin.—Objects of clothing.—Flannel useful under certain circumstances.—Soldiers, and coal heavers on board steamers.—Flannel a bad conductor of heat and cold.—Liability to error from habit.—Stockings.—What kinds are best.—Interesting facts. —Effects of cold bathing in enabling us to do with less clothing.— Spirit drinkers, although they have a warmer surface, suffer more with cold than water drinkers.—Rules in regard to clothing.— Tepid, cool, or cold bathing aids in making a change to lighter clothing.—Caution to the consumptive.—Dr. Combe controverted on the subject of wearing flannel.—The objections to flannel, and its advantages.—Bed clothing.—What it should be.—Evils of cotton comfortables.

ANIMAL sensibility, as affected by heat, cold, and vicissitudes of temperature, is one of the most curious, interesting, and at the same time difficult of all physiological subjects. As in physics, so in physiology, heat and cold are *relative* terms. What is warm and comfortable to the feelings at one time, may be cold and uncomfortable at another; and one person, or one part of a person may be of comfortable temperature, while another, in the same atmosphere, or under the same degree of temperature in surrounding bodies, may experience very different sensations.

The following is an interesting experiment: Temperature of atmosphere 55° F., body of comfortable warmth; took three basins of water at 60, 70, and 80°

F.; placed one hand in the water at 60, the other in that at 80; let them remain thirty seconds, and then placed both hands in the water at 70—to one it was cold, to the other warm.

In a cold winter's morning, if we go from a warm bed to a bath of 65 to 70° F., the water appears cold. If we then plunge into cold water which is at about freezing point, and from that return to the former bath, it appears warm and agreeable to the feelings.

It is said that on a road over the Andes, at about half way between the foot and the summit, there is a cottage in which the ascending and descending travelers meet; the former, who have just quitted the sultry valleys at the base, are so relaxed that the sudden diminution of temperature produces in them a feeling of intense cold; while the latter, who left the frozen summit of the mountain, are overcome by distressing sensations of extreme heat.

Most persons have read the story of the Scythian who went naked about the market-place of Athens, to the great wonder of the people. On being questioned by one of the philosophers how he could go about so naked in the cold, asked in reply, why the other did not cover his face up in winter. Upon the Athenian answering that it was accustomed to the cold, the Scythian rejoined, "Then consider my body as being all face." These familiar facts will serve to throw light on the important subject of clothing as a means of prevention and cure of disease.

I will here remark, that I do not at all agree with those authors who hold that it is *natural* for man to go naked as other animals do. I believe most fully that the human body was created *for* clothing; that the Almighty *intended* that raiment should be worn by human beings : otherwise he would have supplied us with hair, the same as our prototypes, the orang-outang, or monkey kind. Otherwise, too, the universal instinct of the race would not have prompted man to cover the body, as it has done. At the same time, I recognize the important fact that the *amount* of clothing worn should vary as much as the temperatures of the atmosphere in all the different climates that are habitable by man, and also the no less important consideration, that the skin is, to a considerable extent, a *breathing* organ ; and that, as a consequence, the clothing should always be of such character as to admit a constant change of air over its surface. I admit also that the quality and character of clothing are sufficient to cause a great difference in regard to health.

Concerning the use of flannel next to the skin a great deal has been written on the one hand in praise of its effects, and on the other, not a little against it. Some recommend that it be worn continually. Dr. Rush said, that in order to be safe, a person should throw it off one day in the height of summer, and on the next again resume it. Others would have us wear it only in the cool and cold seasons. Others again recommend that it be worn both night and day ; and still others, that we wear it during the day only. We see, too, that some very healthy and hardy persons wear flannel from one end of the year to the other; we see, also. other persons who never wear it at all, and appear equally hardy and robust. How are we to settle these conflicting theories and practices among mankind?

On looking the whole subject over, and analyzing carefully all that the different writers have said both for and against the use of flannel next to the surface, I think it will be plain that there is a much greater *apparent* than *real* difference between the advocates of the two modes. All, I believe, agree in one important point, namely, that in whatever part of the world an individual may be situated, he should be comfortably and agreeably clad. It is to be observed, however, that much more is to be feared from the effects of heat than from the effects of cold.

The objects of clothing, as will be seen from the foregoing remarks, I hold to be—

1. A covering to the body; and,
2. A means of regulating its warmth.

That clothing was designed by our Maker as a *covering* to the body, the natural instincts of all nations prove. Moreover, in the sultry seasons of the tropics it is advantageously used as a *protection from heat*. In the colder regions it is used as a *protection from cold*.

I am willing to admit, or rather, I affirm, that I believe flannel worn next to the skin is often, on the whole, productive of good. Soldiers, who are much exposed to inclemencies of weather and to great changes and vicissitudes of temperature, are no doubt often the better for being warmly clad in woolen garments, even when worn next to the skin. The same may be said of sailors, in the colder parts of the world. Firemen on steamships, and all who are exposed by their occupation to a high degree of heat, from which they must often pass quickly to a colder atmosphere, are also the better for wearing flannel, I have no doubt; still, I believe that in all these cases there is a still better mode.

One of the most important advantages claimed by writers generally for the use of flannel next to the skin, I admit, namely, its power of protecting the body from a too rapid abstraction of its heat. In the language of chemistry, flannel is a bad conductor of caloric; hence the feeling of warmth it causes, and hence its effect as a protection against severe cold. Whenever, then, it is ascertained that the living body is to be subjected to any set of circumstances in which too much of its caloric is liable to be dissipated, the use of flannel is an invaluable means of preserving the health.

But there is great liability to error in whatever pertains to the animal sensations we experience. It is an old saying, that habit becomes use. If a child of healthy instinct has placed in its mouth a piece of tobacco, or a sip of tea, or coffee, or spirits, it instantly rejects each and every one of them as being offensive to the instinct and unfriendly to life. But every one knows, and many to their sad experience, that these natural manifestations of healthy instinct may be readily overcome, and that any substance, however nauseous, deadly, and unfriendly to life it may be in the beginning, may, by frequent and repeated trials, become pleasant and agreeable; nay, more, the individual may feel as if he cannot live without it if he be denied its use.

In applying these physiological principles to the subject of clothing, we at once perceive that there is much liability in regard to the quality and quantity worn. Some men tell us, in this northern country, who have tried the experiment, that their feet are warmer in winter when they go habitually without stockings. Such has been true of lumbermen, who labor constantly in the forest during the winter season. Such has been true, too, of stage-coach drivers and sailors. Now, here we are to infer that habit has much to do in the matter. If the feet are constantly subjected to the more rapid abstraction of caloric, they appear also at the same time to acquire the power of generating more warmth. I myself usually wear linen stockings in the coldest weather. Two years ago, when at Graefenberg, in Germany, while the weather was exceedingly cold—about 10° below zero, F.—I wore thin summer clothing; thin linen pantaloons, without drawers, and at the same time linen stockings. I was, to be sure, quite active in my habits, and took a cold bath daily. I certainly never endured the cold better; and why I mention these facts is this: I have, at times, by way of experiment, exchanged my linen stockings for woolen ones; the effect has been to make my feet colder—that is, colder judging from the sensations produced; and I account for the fact in this way: the linen allowed a free passage of caloric from the skin of the parts, and this going on continually, in connection with the cold bathing which was practiced daily, the surface gained great power of evolving heat. When I put woolen on the feet, I suppose too much caloric was retained upon the surface, so that the difference between its temperature and that of the surrounding air was made greater; in other words, the air about the feet appeared colder than it really was, or greater at least than before. It is to be observed, too, that in all these cases, woolen being thicker than linen, may to some extent prevent circulation by its pressure; but the principal cause of the feeling of coldness which I experienced is, I think, to be explained on the principle to which I have alluded.

I was myself, some years since, very feeble in health. I judge no one can possibly be more sensitive to the unpleasant feeling of cold than I was; but by persevering in cold bathing during one whole cold winter, with Croton water, in the city of New York, and at the same time exercising freely, and living upon a well-selected diet of farinaceous articles and fruits, with a moderate use of milk, I became hardy and strong; and during the second winter of my experiment could endure cold apparently better than ever before in my life. I could then, as I do now, wear the same linen shirts, without under-garments of any kind, without any discomfort the winter through, and, as I believe, with positive good. True, when going from a warm room, I am in the habit of putting on an overcoat or cloak, which is sufficient to protect the body from the cold; but as to my under-garments they are the same the year round, and I wear no woolen whatever, except in the form of external clothing. Now in experience of this kind we see how much habit in subjecting one's surface to the cold has to do in enabling the body to withstand its

effects. That a mere warming of the surface, or increasing the temperature of the body, is of itself not
sufficient to enable it to withstand the effects of cold,
is clearly proved by the fact that spirit drinkers always suffer most, and die soonest, under great exposure to fatigue and cold. Spirit, we know, stimulates
the system; it increases the action of the heart and
arteries, and makes the skin warmer; and notwithstanding it was looked upon, for ages, as being one of
the best means of protecting the living body from severe exposures of this kind, it has been abundantly
proved that water drinkers always endure such hard-
ships better than those who take an opposite course.

The best rules, then, which I can give in regard to
clothing for consumptive persons, as well as others,
are these:

1. Remember always that we are much more liable
to suffer from too great an amount of heat than from
that of cold.

2. That our sensations deceive us on the side of
warmth, and not of cold; in other words, we cannot
acquire the habit of being habitually too cold, without
feeling it; but we may easily acquire the habit of
being too warm, when our sensations do not tell us
that we are so.

3. That soft-spun linen, worn next to the surface,
is, of all substances, the most cleanly, healthful, pleasant, and at the same time most agreeable to the sensations, provided that, in connection, we are properly
shielded from cold.

4. That we should always strive to wear as little
clothing as possible, provided it be, at the same time,

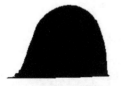

sufficient to guard the system properly against the changes of temperature to which we are subjected.

5. That whatever article is worn next to the surface, the cleaner it is kept, and the oftener aired, the better. We should always change our clothing at least morning and evening of each day. This latter rule is especially applicable to the sick.

I wish here again to enforce the remark, that all changes to the less amount of clothing can be made much more easily in connection with tepid, cool, or cold bathing, managed according to the individual's strength. Tepid water, even, is in fact cooling to the surface, and is, therefore, to be ranked with the cold bath, which is suited to those who are in very feeble health, to consumptive patients in the last stages of the disease, and to all who are greatly debilitated, from whatever cause. The less the strength, let it be remembered, the less cold can be borne.

Consumptive persons, who are in the habit already of wearing woolen next to the surface, should not, as a general thing, especially in the latter stages of the disease, remove it all at once. Put first a linen shirt underneath it, or, if that cannot be had, cotton, which is next best. In some cases, wearing two shirts of linen, or muslin, will be found better than to retain the woolen; but whenever it is necessary let the woolen be retained; only do not let it come next to the skin. Should an individual, at first, feel somewhat colder for putting linen under the woolen, let the skin be well rubbed with the hand, wet in cold water, just before making the change; it will then be easily borne.

The individual may wrap up a little more, externally, at the same time.

Before closing what I have to say on the subject of clothing, I will remark, in regard to that most excellent work, "The Principles of Physiology applied to the Preservation of Health, and to the Importance of Physical and Mental Education"—the author of which, Dr. Andrew Combe, is now no more among the living, and whose work I could wish might be placed in every family that can read—that he has made, I consider, one radical error, in his recommendation of flannel worn next to the skin. Certainly, Doctor Combe was, in general, a most accurate interpreter of the laws of nature; but, in this one thing, he, like many others, was manifestly in error. I admit, as has been seen, his first position, namely, that flannel serves as a protection against cold; but his second position, that, by its stimulation of the cutaneous vessels and nerves of the body, it effects good, I cannot consent to. My reason is this: any thing which acts so continuously upon the system as flannel worn constantly—even though by day only—must soon lose its effect. If we were to wear the flannel an hour or two at a time, once or twice during the day, this excitation of the surface might, I am willing to admit, accomplish good, especially with those who are not in the habit of bathing, and keeping themselves clean; but to apply this process continually, it must necessarily lose its effects.

There is also another way in which flannel may injure, and which should not be forgotten. If a person goes into the open air, when it is cold, he needs a certain amount of clothing; when he passes into a warm room, to remain, all will agree, I think, that he needs less flannel. We are to believe, then, that flannel, although good when we go out, must be not only unnecessary, but positively injurious, by its causing too great warmth, when we are within doors.

There is yet another important practical fact connected with a change of temperature, which should be particularly remembered by those who have any form of ulceration in the lungs. It is this—too great exposure to cold, or too much cooling of the system by any means, tends certainly to hasten the process of ulceration. Any thing, then, whether in changes of clothing, bathing, or climate, or any change which robs the system of too great an amount of heat, is positively detrimental in the latter stages of pulmonary consumption, as also in any disease whatever where extensive ulceration exists.

The objections to which flannel is liable, stated briefly, are as follows:

1. It is too great an irritant to the skin, more especially if the article be not very fine.

2. It aggravates cutaneous eruptions, and when these are already present it prevents their cure.

3. It causes too great heat of the immediate surface of the skin, thereby weakening it and rendering it more sensitive to the impression of wet and cold.

4. It promotes an undue degree of perspiration, thereby debilitating the skin, and through it the whole system.

The advantages of flannel are:

1. That it affords a protection against cold.

2. That possibly, in a very hot day, or in any case where a person perspires much, it may be a more agreeable article to the feelings, as when moist or wet it admits more air to the surface than linen or cotton would do.

Bed clothing.—It is proper that a few words should here be said on this subject. There is one custom which is very prevalent at the present day in our country, and which should be strongly reprobated. I refer to the use of cotton comfortables. These act injuriously in two ways. They retain too much heat about the surface of the body, and at the same time the cutaneous emanations are not allowed sufficiently to pass off. Woolen blankets outside of the sheets are, in all respects, much preferable to cotton comfortables, and articles of similar kind.

Most persons use too great an amount of covering at night. The same general rules hold good here, as in regard to the clothing worn by day. We should always use as little as possible, which is, at the same time, sufficient to fulfill all the good objects for which clothing is designed.

THE END.

INDEX.

THE

WATER-CURE

IN

PREGNANCY AND CHILDBIRTH,

Illustrated with Cases,

SHOWING THE

REMARKABLE EFFECTS OF WATER

IN

MITIGATING THE PAINS AND PERILS

OF THE

PARTURIENT STATE.

BY JOEL SHEW, M.D.

STEREOTYPED

—

NEW YORK:

FOWLERS & WELLS, PUBLISHERS,

NO. 308 BROADWAY.

In Boston:
142 Washington Street.

1855.

Philadelphia:
No. 231 Arch Street.

PREFACE.

It is said that in China, the practice of midwifery is regulated in this wise : Female midwives attend in all the ordinary cases; but there is a class of obstetric surgeons, devoted exclusively to this department, perfectly skilled in the use of instruments, and the management of every possible difficulty. One of these is located in a particular district, with a given number of inhabitants, and after a woman has been a certain number of hours in labor, the midwife is required by law to call in the surgeon. Now I hold that an arrangement similar to this ought to exist in every civilized and enlightened country. Women should, for the most part, be the practitioners of midwifery. This is so obviously true that it needs no argument. I do not wish, then, to conceal the fact, that this work has been written with the view of doing somewhat, however small it may be, toward the prevention of the almost universal custom of employing man-midwives in this country at the present day.

But, as will be easily seen, this work does not profess to teach the *art* of midwifery. It presupposes, as far as the time of labor is concerned, that the attendant, male or female, has already a knowledge of the science pertaining to this department. My main design has been to show how water may be applied as a great and universal tonic in pregnancy and childbirth. These directions, if skillfully and faithfully carried out, will be found the sure means of producing an amount of benefit and relief that can only be conceived of by those who are brought actually to experience them.

Within a few years past, persons have often written me from a distance, that they had followed the advice as laid down, from time to time, in the Water-Cure Journal, for females at the times of pregnancy and childbirth, and that they had experienced the great-

eat benefit by so doing.   Persons have said, "I had borne a number of children previously, suffering at each time more than tongue
can describe; and now since I have been under the water-treatment, the whole matter has been reduced to a comparatively trifling affair."   I am convinced, therefore, that this work, small as it
is, will be the means of greatly mitigating the pains and sufferings
of many who will deign to follow its advice.

There is one circumstance which, in our country, is eminently
calculated to keep back reform in midwifery matters.   We have
every where about three times as many physicians as are necessary to do even what is done; and there is a great deal more *doc-
toring* than need be, as every one knows.   Midwifery practice is
one of the most profitable branches of the medical art.   Can we
suppose, then, that medical men, a majority of whom have hard
work "to keep body and soul together," will allow old women to
take from them the very bread they eat?   Never, so long as by any
possibility they can prevent it.   But there is encouragement in the
matter.   People are beginning more and more to read, think, and
act, for themselves.   Medical men, may persist in denouncing cold
water, yet there are those who *will* resort to it, and from a *knowledge* of its efficacy.   J. S.

New York, 1849.

CONTENTS

CHAPTER I.

USES OF WATER INTERNALLY 11–24

Water the best of all Drinks.—Composition of the Human Body.—The Living Body compared to a Furnace.—Drinking in Fevers.—Does Man naturally Drink ?—Danger of Drinking when Fatigued.—Rules for Water-Drinking.—Drinking at Meals.—Water does not dilute the Gastric Juice.—Thirst not common when the Dietetic Habits are good.—Water-Drinking good in Acid Stomach and Heart-burn.—Wind in the Stomach.—Water in Cholera.—Common Water better than Mineral.—Water in Headache.—Nausea in Pregnancy.—Good effects of Water-Vomiting.—Harsh means not allowable in Pregnancy.—Water-Drinking in Palpitation of the Heart.—It increases the Milk.—Clysters or Injections.—These are much better than Cathartic Medicines.—Rules for their Use.—Good in Loosenesses of the Bowels as well as in Constipation.—Also in Colics.—Their use in Childbirth.—Uterine Hæmorrhage.—Fainting Fits and Hysteria.—Cholera Infantum.—Affections of the Urinary Passages.—Piles and Hæmorrhoids.

CHAPTER II.

MODES OF BATHING 25–44

The rubbing Wet-Sheet.—Dr. Graham Controverted.—The Towel Bath.—Sponge Bath.—Bath by Affusion.—Plunge Bath.—Shower Bath.—How it is to be Used.—Douche Bath.—Its Uses.—A Small Douche milder than the Shower.—Half Bath.—Its various Effects.—Head Bath.—Conditions in which it is Useful.—Nasal Bath.—An excellent Remedy in Colds.—Oral or Mouth Bath and its Uses.—Sitz or Hip Bath.—Invaluable in Pregnancy.—Cold Foot Bath.—Erroneous Notions concerning its Use.—Good for a variety of Purposes.—Warm Foot Bath.—General Directions concerning Baths.—How often should we Bathe ?

CHAPTER III.

COMPRESSES OR BANDAGES, AND THE WET SHEET, 45–54

Wet Compresses or Bandages Important Means of Water-Cure.—Cooling Compresses.—The Warming or Stimulating.—The Soothing.—Warm and Hot Fomentations.—The Wet Girdle.—Its Mode of Application and Uses.—Oil and India Rubber Cloth Bandages.—The German Water Dressing for Wounds, Cuts, etc.—The Wet Sheet.—Mode of Applying it.—Its Soothing Effects.—Not to be Used for Sweating.—Bathing after the Sheet.—Wet Sheets in Fevers and Inflammations.—Becoming Cold in the Wet Sheet.—Heat and Fullness in the Head.—The Wet Sheet applicable in Pregnancy.

CHAPTER IV.

DISORDERS OF PREGNANCY 55–69

Febrile Condition of the System during the period of Pregnancy.—This may be greatly Modified by Diet, and general Regimen.—Protecting Power of Pregnancy.—Diseased Persons should not Procreate.—Acute Diseases more dangerous in Pregnancy.—Harsh Means not allowable during this Period. —Insomnia or Sleeplessness in Pregnancy.—How to be Prevented.—Headache.—Sometimes a dangerous Symptom in Pregnancy.—The Remedial Means.—Sick or Nervous Headache.—Tea and Coffee often Causes of this Disease.—Breeding with a Toothache.—How to be Remedied.—Teeth not to be Extracted during Pregnancy.—Salivation.—This is often a Troublesome Complaint.—How it is to be Remedied.—Difficulty in Breathing.—Heart-Burn.—Too much Food generally a Cause.—Means of Preventing it.

CHAPTER V.

Nausea and Vomiting.—These Symptoms more common in the early months of Pregnancy.—What Persons are most subject to them.—Vomiting sometimes becomes Dangerous.—How Nausea and Vomiting are to be Prevented.—Morbid Craving or Longing for particular articles of food in Pregnancy.—These should not be gratified.—Pain in the Right Side.—How to be Remedied.—Constipation.—This is most common in the earlier months of Gestation.—Causes of Constipation.—Remedial Means to be Used.—These the same as in Constipation ordinarily.—Diarrhœa in Pregnancy.—Not so frequent as Constipation.—Both to be treated on the same General Principles.—Piles and Hæmorrhoids.—Modes of Treatment.—Difficulty of voiding Urine.—How to be Remedied.—Itching of the Genital Parts.—Water a sovereign Remedy.—Swelling of the Limbs.—Varicose Veins.—Cramps in the Lower Extremities.—Pain in the Breasts.—How to be treated.—Warm or hot Applications sometimes Useful.—The Mind as affected by Pregnancy.—Women are more apt to become irritable at this time.—Hysteria in Pregnancy.

CHAPTER VI.

Miscarriage or Abortion becoming more common at the present day.—The reasons why.—Rules to be Observed.—What Females are most liable to Abortion.—Vile Books concerning Abortion.—Means of Preventing it.—Cold Water an excellent Remedy.—Feather Beds and Pillows injurious.—Vegetable Diet better than Animal.—Hæmorrhage from the womb in Pregnancy not necessarily attended with Abortion—Abortion generally a more serious matter than Labor at full term.—Those who miscarry once are more apt to do so again.—Very feeble Persons should not become Pregnant.—The treatment in Miscarriage.—What to do in the absence of a Physician.—Cold a better means than Blood-letting for arresting Uterine Hæmorrhage.—Barrenness.—Bathing and Diet often effectual in this matter.

CHAPTER VII.

CHAPTER VIII.

Management after Childbirth.—Popular objections answered.—The evils of Confinement in Bed.—The injurious Effects of the common Bandage or Binder.—The use of cold Water and the wet Girdle in all respects better Means.—After-Pains.—How to be prevented.—Swelling of the Breasts.—Cold Water a sovereign Remedy.—Sore Nipples.—Injections after Labor.—Management of the Child.—When to separate the Umbilical Cord.—The best mode of washing the Infant.—The common Bandage not to be Applied.—Very important Advice as regards weaning and feeding Infants.

WATER-CURE
IN
PREGNANCY AND CHILDBIRTH.

CHAPTER I.

USES OF WATER INTERNALLY.*

Water the best of all Drinks.—Composition of the Human Body.—The Living Body compared to a Furnace.—Drinking in Fevers.—Does Man naturally Drink ?—Danger of Drinking when Fatigued.—Rules for Water-Drinking.—Drinking at Meals.—Water does not dilute the Gastric Juice.—Thirst not common when the Dietetic Habits are good.—Water-Drinking good in Acid Stomach and Heart-burn.—Wind in the Stomach.—Water in Cholera.—Common Water better than Mineral.—Water in Headache.—Nausea in Pregnancy.—Good effects of Water-Vomiting.—Harsh means not allowable in Pregnancy.—Water-Drinking in Palpitation of the Heart.—It increases the Milk.—Clysters or Injections.—These are much better than Cathartic Medicines.—Rules for their Use.—Good in Looseinesses of the Bowels as well as in Constipation.—Also in Colics.—Their use in Childbirth.—Uterine Hæmorrhage.—Fainting Fits and Hysteria.—Cholera Infantum.—Affections of the Urinary Passages.—Piles and Hæmorrhoids.

WATER is the best of all drinks ; the best to promote healthfulness of body, vigor, cheerfulness, and contentment of the mind ; the best to enable the system to endure excessive heat, cold, or protracted exertion of any of the faculties of man. How different from this universally received opinion has been the practice of ages !

* It is to be presumed, that this work will fall into the hands of many who are not informed on the subject of the " Processes of the Water-Cure ;" and for this reason the author has deemed it necessary here to give a short explanation of the modes of using water, as applicable generally, as well as in the conditions of Pregnancy and Childbirth. These are, in part, compiled from the Water-Cure Manual, to which the reader is referred for a still more full account of the water modes.

Immediately after the flood, it was found that he who was chosen above all others as the favored of Heaven, had yet within him the artificial love for intoxicating substances ; and how far back in the period of man's history these substances were used, it would be difficult, if not impossible, to determine.

It has been a question with some whether man is *naturally* a drinking animal. One author of notoriety, Dr. Lambe, argues that we must suppose every animal to be furnished with organs suited to its physical necessities. "Now I see," continues this writer, "that man has the head elevated above the ground, and to bring the mouth to the earth, requires a strained and painful effort. Moreover, the mouth is flat and the nose prominent, circumstances which make the effort still more difficult." But in all this reasoning, it is forgotten that one of the most pleasant, safe, and natural modes of drinking water, is that from the hand. If a person is wandering of a sultry summer day, along the mountain side, and parched and thirsty, and comes to a spring, pure, fresh, and bubbling, he very quickly lifts the fluid portion by portion, in the half-closed hand, and raises it to his lips ; besides, it is as natural for man to employ his ingenuity, provided this is done in accordance with certain laws, as for animals instinct. Man, I have no doubt, like animals, in general, drinks.

The human body, as a whole, by weight, consists of about 80 parts, in the 100, of water. Even its dryer portions, as bone, muscle, cartilage, ligament, and nerve, contain a large proportion of this fluid. The blood has about 90 parts, in the 100, and the brain nearly the same proportion. Without the presence of water in the living body, food would not become digested in the stomach ;

no chyme would be elaborated to supply the chyle, or chyle to form the blood. Respiration, circulation, secretion, nutrition, perspiration, elimination—neither of these could take place in the human system, without the presence of a large proportion of water.

The living body may be compared to a perpetual furnace, which has a tendency, constantly, by evaporation, to become dry. If food and water are, in every form, withheld, the individual grows parched and feverish. In a few days, delirium supervenes, and, in about three weeks, he dies. But if water be taken according to the demands of thirst, no fever or delirium ensue, and life goes on more than twice as long as when both food and drink are withheld. From these considerations, it is evident that the living body must be frequently supplied with a considerable amount of water.

Shall we drink in fevers and inflammatory diseases? We can scarcely give a lecture, enter a neighborhood, or even a family, and introduce the subject of water, but that we are at once told of remarkable instances of cure, which the narrator has known to take place through the drinking of water. The patient was very sick; learned physicians declared, " For his life he must not touch cold water." Every thing fails; the man grows worse—is given up; and, in the long, dark night, to give some small relief from his raging thirst, water is administered. The friends tremble for his safety, but he appears to grow better, and more is given. Sleep and perspiration ensue. The patient lives, " *in spite of cold water*," shall any one say? Or, perhaps, in his delirium, he has broken over all bonds, and quaffed, suddenly and deep, of the fluid which, above all earthly things, he craved; or, by stealth, hire, or threats, he ac-

2

complishes his object.   Whoever knew a patient in high,
burning fever (not induced by over-exertion), killed by
cold water?   Many have been thus saved, but more,
alas! incomparably more, have been lost, for the want
of its use.

Let the sick drink freely, copiously, according to the
demands of thirst.   Be the disease curable or fatal, deny
it not.   Even in the last hours of consumption, by
draughts of pure cold water, let the fever be quelled, the
suffering mitigated, and every thing done possible that
may be, to smooth, in some degree, however small, the
sufferer's passage to the grave.

Every one is well aware, that life is sometimes suddenly destroyed by persons drinking a large quantity
of cold water when greatly fatigued.   It is easy to avoid
all danger in these cases, by sipping the water, only a
few drops at a time, as it were.   The body is already in
perspiration, which is, of itself, a cooling process; and
a small quantity of water, slowly taken, proves sufficient,
soon, to quench the thirst.   Washing the face, hands,
and temples, and holding water in the mouth, are safe
and excellent means.

A very good rule for the healthy, and such as have
active exercise, is to drink, except in fatigue and exhaustion, as thirst demands.   Patients may have the
general direction to take at such times, as when the
stomach is empty, as much as can be conveniently
borne, which will generally be from six to twelve half-
pint tumblers in the whole day.   Feeble persons must
not go on very rapidly at first.   If they have been accustomed a long time to hot drinks, they should, on commencing, make small beginnings, gradually training the
stomach in the new way.   Wonders may thus be ac-

complished, if the patient can have system and perseverance enough to proceed.

The better statement for invalids, perhaps, is "exercise as much as may be without causing too great fatigue ; by this means, the system becomes invigorated and warmed ; more fluid is thrown off, more is needed, and more relished ; so exercise and drink as much as you conveniently can." The water should, if possible, always be pure and soft.

People generally have an impression, that drinking at meals is injurious ; and yet they are ready enough to take soups, tea, coffee, cocoa, chocolate, and the like, not to mention stronger articles, healthy or unhealthy, as fluids may be. It is said the gastric juice is diluted and weakened, and that therefore digestion is retarded. But it should be understood that the stomach is not a sack for holding gastric juice. The first part of digestion is the absorption of the more fluid portion of the food. The more solid contents are crowded to the lower or pyloric part of the stomach, and a sort of hour-glass contraction takes place. The fluid becomes absorbed, and afterward, as the churn-like motion of the stomach commences, the gastric juice oozes forth like perspiration upon the surface, to commingle with the food. Does not every one know that grapes, apples, and the like substances, almost all water, are among the most healthful forms of food ? In fact, these substances, taken in suitable quantity, as by half tea-spoon doses, if the stomach is so weak as to require that, are, to say the least, among the very best things possible for the sick. This is especially true in fevers, in which cases food is so illy borne ; and certainly, food that is good for the sick must be as good for the well, needed of course in greater quantity, proportioned to the amount of strength. It is a question with some physiologists whether drinking should be practiced at all with the meals. Certainly it cannot be bad to drink with the food for the reason generally assigned, namely, because water dilutes the gastric juice. But water is absorbed from the stomach before the gastric begins to flow. Therefore the objection cannot prove good. Farmers, and those who labor much during the long, hot days of summer, sweating a great deal, as they must necessarily do, tell us that if they drink freely at meal-times, they need much less water, or, in other words, experience much less thirst. Here then would seem to be an argument in favor of drinking at meals. Almost every kind of food is made up, the larger part, of water. Even baker's bread contains 35 per cent. ; domestic bread generally more than 50 per cent.

If all the habits are well regulated, true natural thirst will seldom be experienced by the healthy, and it remains yet to be proved, that (except in certain cases, as in hickup, heart-burn, acidity, etc.) the drinking of water is useful at such times as when there is no thirst.

Some have fallen into the error of advocating the disuse of drink in acidity, heart-burn, and the like. Generally in such cases there is no thirst, but sometimes this becomes very tormenting. Now in all these cases, if I can understand the effects of water, both upon myself and others, I am certain that copious drinking is one of the best, if not *the* best, means that can be used, *i. e.*, after the difficulty is already present. Better much, of course, to avoid the trouble by practicing sufficient moderation in food, but if the evil comes, drink until relief is experienced.

Digestion is one thing and fermentation another, and very different. If the stomach is weak, food is apt to pass at once into acetous fermentation, just as would be were it in any other warm, moist place. The acid substance is an irritant or excitant to the coats of the organ, thus causing the difficulties in question. The more it is diluted, therefore, the less effect can it have, and the sooner is it washed away. The undue heat in the part is quelled, and the stomach is invigorated, the better to perform its functions.

Wind upon the stomach may be expelled by drinking very often small quantities of water. This advice, if followed, will prove useful often in pregnancy.

The smaller difficulties of digestion had perhaps better not be interfered with. When the process goes on fairly, three or more hours should supervene before drinking is commenced. Toward the end of digestion, the stomach becomes jaded, so to speak, when the sipping of water will prove salutary.

It is a fashion for the profession to assert that nothing is known of the true mode of treating the cholera, because the opinions concerning it were so contradictory. It has been ascertained, that one of the best modes of treating this dreadful disease is to give the patient as much ice and ice-water as he desires; and it is astonishing what quantities cholera patients will take. There is no disease in which the serum or watery part of the blood passes off so rapidly as in this. There must necessarily be a thirst proportioned to the loss of fluid, and there is no other disease in which such enormous quantities of water are tolerated as in this.

Constipation often occurs in pregnancy. Persons are always bettered more or less in this complaint by drink-

2*

ing freely of pure soft water. Nothing, however, will answer fully for plainness of food in these cases. Patients go to watering-places, leave their cares, anxieties, excessive labors, mental and physical, rise early, go much in the open air, drink spring water, and by so doing are sometimes benefited, sometimes made worse. The same principle precisely holds good in the use of all mineral waters as in drugs. It is for the *drug* effects only that they are taken. The same amount of pure soft water, drank in connection with the other favorable circumstances, would be incomparably better than the mineral water. Ask one hundred persons who have tried both methods, and ninety-nine, if not the whole number, will decide in accordance with that which I have affirmed. An old English author says, that a patient found that his own pump water did as much good as the Bristol waters, where he had been the summer before, whereupon he wrote—

> " The steel is a cheat,
> 'Tis water does the feat."

Many persons troubled with headache, have only to restrict themselves to water-drinking, partaking temperately of plain food, and the difficulty vanishes. This advice will do well for many persons who are not pregnant, as well as those who are.

In the nausea of pregnancy, the drinking freely of pure soft water will be found very serviceable. And if there is need of an emetic, as in internal cramps, colics, pain in the bowels, flatulency, prostration by heat or cold, poisoning, etc., water-vomiting is a most serviceable means. Drink many tumblers of blood-warm water, place the finger in the throat, or knead the stomach, and the vomiting ensues. Repeat the process again and again, till the organ is completely cleansed. Perseverance must be practiced here, in some cases, at least. Persons must be urged to the work, if they have not, of themselves, courage enough. The sick cannot always be their own masters in these things. If a cathartic action is caused by the water drank, the effect is good. Harsh means are of course never allowable in pregnancy, because of the danger of abortion. But the vomiting by water is so easy, and attended with so little retching, it may safely be practiced whenever there is need.

PALPITATION OF THE HEART.

A common symptom at all times among females who drink strong tea and coffee, and which is also still more common in pregnancy, will, in many cases, be cured merely by coming down to the cold-water plan, and excluding all other drinks. In many cases this desirable result will be obtained in a very short time ; in other cases, weeks, or even months, may be required. Sick headaches, which are, in multitudes of cases, only tea and coffee headaches, come also under this rule.

Pure soft water increases the milk of nursing mothers when the secretion is scant. An old English writer on water, says : " By divers experiments it hath been found true, that the drinking of water by nurses while they give suck to children, will wonderfully increase milk in those that want it, as every one will find who can be persuaded to make use thereof. I have advised many to make use of it, who have found that by drinking a large draught of water at bed-time, they have been supplied with milk sufficient for that night, when before they wanted it, and could not be supplied by any other means; and besides, they who have found their children restless, by reason of too much heat in their milk, do find them much more quiet after their milk is cooled by water-drinking."*

THE ENEMA, CLYSTER, OR INJECTION.

This very important part of the water-cure is as old as the healing art itself, but in the endless complications of the remedial means of modern times, almost any irritating or disgusting fluid, other than pure water, is preferred. A variety of instruments for administering injections are now manufactured, varying in price from fifty cents to four or five dollars. The cheaper kinds, if well made and used with some degree of dexterity, answer a good purpose. Every person should have access to one; no lady's toilet is complete without it. Contrary to the common notion, a person, by the exercise of a little skill, can easily use this remedy without assistance. It is in no wise painful, but decidedly agreeable, and affords, in a variety of complaints, speedy and efficient relief. Thousands suffer incalculably from constipation, year after year, when the use of this simple means would give the greatest relief, and thousands more are in the daily and constant habit of swallowing cathartic and aperient drugs, Brandreth's pills, castor oil, magnesia, blue pill, mercury, and so through the long chapter, that irritate and poison the delicate coats of the stomach, and exert their pernicious influence

---

* Curiosities of Common Water. By John Smith, C. M. 1723. A very instructive work, lately republished by Fowlers & Wells, New York.

throughout the numberless lanes and alleys of the system, destroying the healthy tone of the tissues, deranging the nerves, and thus causing a state of things incomparably worse than the disease itself, and rendering even that more and more persistent.

Most persons may and should use this remedy cold. A beginning may be made with the water slightly warmed. In obstinate cases, luke-warm water effects the object quicker and with greater certainty than cold. It may be repeated again and again, in as great quantity as is desired. Some prefer the clyster before breakfast; others immediately after; the former, I believe, on the whole, to be the best. A good mode, too, is to take a small injection, a tumbler full, more or less, that is retained permanently without a movement before morning. This is very soothing to the nervous system, aids in procuring sound sleep, and by its absorption in the coats of the bowels, dilutes acrid matters therein, tonifying and strengthening likewise those parts, and aiding materially in bringing about natural movements; but invaluable and efficient as is this remedy, let no one persist in those habits of diet, such as tea and coffee drinking, the use of heating and stimulating condiments, greasy and concentrated forms of food, etc., that tend so certainly to constipation and irregularity of the bowels.

In all forms of looseness of the bowels, as diarrhœa, dysentery, cholera morbus, cholera infantum, and the like, this remedy is most excellent. In many a sudden attack, injections, sufficiently persevered in, will suffice quickly to correct the attack, and this when, in the ordinary treatment, a course of powerful drugging would be deemed indispensable, that would result perhaps in

death.   This statement will cause sneering, I know, but
it is no fancy sketch.   The thoroughly washing out, so
to say, the lower bowels ; by which also the peristaltic
or downward action of the whole alimentary canal is
promoted, and by the absorption or transudation of water, its contents are moistened and diluted, and the
whole of the abdominal circulation completely suffused,
by that blandest and most soothing of all fluids, pure
water.   I say all this is sufficient to effect, in all such
cases, a great amount of good : and whoever understands well the sympathies and tendencies of these parts
of the human system, will at once perceive the truth of
that I affirm.   So also in constipation and obstructions
of the bowels ; when no powerful cathartics that any
one dare venture to exhibit, can be made to act, this
simple remedy is effectual in bringing about the desirable object.

In any of these cases, if there is debility, and especially if it be great, whether the patient be young or
old, the water should be used of a moderate temperature—not above that of the blood (98 degrees Fah.),
nor very much below that point.   Even if there is high
inflammation and much heat in the bowels, water at 90
or 95 degrees, persevered in, will readily bring down
the temperature of the parts to a natural state, as may
be determined by placing the hand upon the abdomen.
The patient's feelings of comfort as to warmth or cold
are a good guide.   With these precautions as to temperature, etc., the injections may be repeated for an
hour, or even hours upon the stretch.

In attacks of colic, clysters are used much.   In spasmodic colic, I believe, it will generally be found best to
use them quite warm.   In wind colic, the enema is highly

useful. Vomiting as well, and some other means, as is shown elsewhere, should be brought to bear. Some cases are very obstinate, and require all the skill of the most experienced practitioner; yet I advise all persons to persevere; in bad cases, you cannot make matters worse, and will generally succeed if you do not falter by the way.

At the beginning of labor in childbirth, it is advisable that the colon or lower bowel be cleared of its contents. There is generally more or less constipation then; and it is the common practice to administer some cathartic, slow in its operation, and irritating and debilitating in its effects.

The injection is quick and harmless in its action, and always aids, in a greater or less degree, the natural pains in accouchement. It is also invaluable day by day, when needed, after the birth.

In uterine hæmorrhage, or bleeding from the womb, very cold injections might be brought well to bear, but they have seldom if ever been used for that purpose.

In the untold sufferings of painful menstruation, experienced by so many of the fair ones of our country, now-a-days, injections to the bowels are invaluable. Generally chilling cold ones are best here. They do not arrest the menstrual discharge, as would generally be feared, but on the contrary, promote it if too scanty, or check it if too great. If in any case the cold application increases the pain, the warm one is indicated.

In fainting fits, and in hysterical symptoms, the injection is serviceable. If there is much debility, care must be taken that the temperature is not too cold; but, generally, the colder it is given, the better.

In cases of cholera infantum, when the infant is already

past recovery, I have known tepid injections, frequently repeated, give, apparently, much relief; and it affords satisfaction, when nothing more can be done, to be the means, in some degree, of smoothing the passage of these innocent sufferers to the tomb.

Injections to the urinary passages, and to the vagina and womb, are useful in all acute and chronic affections of these parts. The water should generally be used cold. Various instruments are constructed for these purposes.

Piles and hæmorrhoids are more apt to occur in pregnancy than at other times. In all such cases cold injections are indicated. Recent attacks are often cured with wonderful rapidity; and, in any case, those who have been long troubled with these complaints (and it would seem that about one half the number of adults, who lead a sedentary life, are thus troubled), will find, that simple, pure water is incomparably better than any of the thousand-and-one nostrums so much in vogue at this day.

CHAPTER II

MODES OF BATHING.

RUBBING WET-SHEET.

THIS is one of the mildest and most convenient forms
of a bath. A large linen sheet, of coarse material, is
wrung out in cold water, and, while dripping, one or
more assistants immediately aid in rubbing over the
whole surface. Rub over the sheet; not *with* it. This
is continued, briskly, three, five, or more minutes, until
the skin becomes reddened, and the surface in a glow.
The system is then made dry with towels, or a dry
sheet. Frictions with the dry hand, are also very useful. If the patient is feverish, much friction is not required. The sheet is repeated often in such cases.

In determination of blood to the head, the lower extremities being generally cold, the rubbing-sheet tends
to restore an equilibrium of the circulation. The rubbing wet-sheet, in principle, is easily administered to
patients in such a state of health as to render it necessary for them to remain in bed. The person lays upon

3

a blanket, that may be afterward removed : a portion
of the system is rubbed, first with wet towels, followed
with the dry.   This part is then covered, and the other
extremities disposed of in the same way.   The water
should be moderated, according to the strength of the
patient.   All who are able to walk about, to insure
warmth, should take the water cold.

Dr. R. H. Graham, of London, who advocates, strongly the uses of water, but objects to Priessnitz as a practitioner, commits an error in saying, " A glass of water
must be drank immediately before, during, or after this
application, according to the inclination of the patient."
Before no cold bath, whatever, should cold water be
drank.   Even if there is fever and thirst, we should
avoid drinking it.   Most persons may bear such a practice ; but, even with the most robust, the physiological
action of the bath is more beneficial with the drinking
omitted until after it : and then, water should not be
taken internally, until the system becomes decidedly
warm.

Again, Dr. G. says, " It may, moreover, be used immediately after dinner, and with much advantage, when
the body is covered with perspiration, from exercise."
Here, again, is wrong teaching.   Physiology says, unequivocally, " When digestion is going on, take no form,
whatever, of general bath."   If you exercise the muscular system violently, or set the brain hard at work,
the blood and vital power needed at the stomach, is
withdrawn to other parts, and, therefore, it cannot well
do its office ; and if you commence operating upon the
skin, that greatest organ of the system, you, by sympathy, arrest the progress of its work.   I admit, certainly,
that if the dinner has been such (and there are some

who take of this kind) as to throw the system into a decided general fever, this should, by some means, be reduced. Digestion does not now go on. Under such circumstances, then, a person may take the rubbing sheet, or, if strong, almost any form of bath. If it be the fever caused by strong drink, he may lay himself in a tepid bath, and sleep, even, until his fever is removed, and he awakes refreshed. But such modes are very wrong for the well, or those in chronic disease.

As to the other part of Dr. G.'s last statement, if a person is very much fatigued, and covered with perspiration, he must be careful how he meddles with the cold bath. But, if the fatigue has not gone too far, although there is perspiration, the rubbing wet-sheet is one of the most soothing, and, at the same time, invigorating modes that can possibly be found. Such as have become exhausted, from public speaking, strong mental efforts, watchings, and the like, are greatly benefited by the rubbing wet-sheet. If, at any time, the surface is cool, dry frictions or exercise are to be practiced, to induce warmth, before it is used. If a person, from debility, fails of becoming warm, he is well wrapped in dry blankets, a half hour, or more, and, when sufficiently comfortable, the rubbing sheet is again given, to promote the strength. Frictions, with the dry, warm hands of assistants, are always good, in these cases, to help to insure warmth. If a person finds himself remaining cold in the lein-tuch, he should omit that, until the use of the abreibung, exercise, etc., enables him to get warm. The tonic effect of the rubbing sheet is most serviceable in night perspirations and debilitating sweats.

The very soothing effects of the rubbing sheet should

not be lost sight of. In cares, watchings, and in grief this remedy of Priessnitz's is unparalleled in its effects In delirium tremens, and in inebriation, it is most valuable in its results. The rubbing wet-sheet being one of the mildest of all the water processes, as well as one of the most convenient, is particularly applicable in pregnancy.

TOWEL BATH.

By means of wet towels, we may take, almost any where, a good bath. With a single quart of water, we can do this, even in a room, carpeted ever so nice, without spilling a single drop. The towel bath may seem a small matter; but we find none, but the most lazy, who, once accustomed, are willing to relinquish its use. Small matters, oft repeated, and long continued, accomplish much. A *little* medicine is taken, day by day, and at length health fails, and death is the result. Tea, coffee, tobacco, wine, etc., are used in very *small* quantities, and the teeth become dark, and decay; the head aches, the hand trembles, and the spirits fail. So good influences, however small, in the end, accomplish great results.

How can it be, asks an objector, that trifling applications, made externally, become, to the internal organs, so serviceable as some assert? This query may be well answered in the sarcastic words of a good old English writer on water, Dr. Baynard: "A demi-brained doctor, of more note than sense, asked, in the amazed agony of his half-understanding, how 'twas possible that an external application should affect the bowels, and cure the pain within. Why, doctor, quoth an old woman, standing by, by the same reason, that being wet-

shod, or catching cold from without shou.d give you the gripes and pain within."

SPONGE BATH.

Some like to stand in a tub, and use a large sponge, out of which the water is pressed, and made to pass upon the head, neck, and shoulders, and other parts. We may pour water from a cup, basin, or pitcher, if we choose. There appears to be no particular advantage in the sponges; the water is what we need

BATH BY AFFUSION.

A person may stand in a wash-tub or any convenient place, and by means of a pitcher, cup, or hand-basin, pour water upon the neck and shoulders, and thus take a very excellent bath. This simple way will indeed be found, as a general thing, better than the portable shower baths. These are very apt to get out of order, although some of them are very good.

Fifty years ago, Dr. Currie, of England, performed wonders by the affusion of cool and tepid water, graduated in temperature according to the strength of the constitution. In all the varieties of fever he adopted the mode; so in small-pox, measles, scarlatina, as well as in convulsive diseases and in insanity. It is now acknowledged by the highest authority in that country, that Dr. Currie's mode was attended with greater success than any other previously known.

The bath by affusion is a very excellen one to be used in pregnancy. It is not best to take it very cold during this time.

3*

PLUNGE BATH.

In sea, river, and lake, as well as by artificial means, bathing and general ablutions have been practiced from time immemorial; as a matter of luxury, religious observance, purification, prevention, and cure of disease, bathing has been resorted to in every period of the world. So efficacious has this simple means proved in the healing of the sick, that not a little superstition has been mingled with it. Springs and wells have often been supposed to possess some mysterious power, and have, therefore, been named after some pattern saint. The world has loved mystery and marvelousness, and has ever been wandering from simplicity and truth. The plunge bath is not, as a general fact, the best for persons in pregnancy. The rubbing sheet affusions and washings, being milder modes, are better.

THE SHOWER BATH.

This is often wrongly used. As physicians are becoming generally more impressed with the importance of water, they not unfrequently say to a patient, "Take the shower bath." The patient, a lady, perhaps, is very weak. Medicine enough to make her so, quite likely, has been given, and a good bill run up. Last of all, the order comes, "Take the shower bath:" about as philosophic a prescription, as to say to a person in severe constipation, and not at all acquainted with the doses of medicine, "Take Croton oil." Of this most powerful of all purgatives, every one would, of course, take too much. Within three years, since baths are getting to be the fashion, I have known a number of persons materially injured, in consequence of this oose kind of advice.' A great many patients are too weak to take the cold shower bath. Milder means must be used.

The shower bath should never be taken upon the head. Some can bear it; but, in all cases, it is better to wash the part. The head should never be beaten by water, or any thing else. Most men have an idea that taking it upon the head is necessary, to prevent rushing of blood to the part. Cooling the head is, of course, good for this, and, if the bath has but little force, the head is, in many instances, benefited. But it may be beneficially acted upon indirectly, as by the foot bath, which is so good to relieve headache. The hip bath is easily managed, so as to cause the same effect. So, also, the shower bath, upon any or all parts of the body, but the head, may be made to cause the same result. Now the blood at the feet is cooled, and now it has arrived at the head. The blood is rapidly coursing through the system; and thus, by cooling it, we very soon affect the most distant part.

If the person has strength enough, and does not take the shower bath upon the head, he will find no difficulty in its use. It is a very valuable and convenient mode; and many persons have, by this simple means, been most wonderfully restored. And yet some water-practitioners are so prejudiced, that; if a patient commences telling them the benefit he has derived from its use, they at once fall into a rage. It is easy, in these cases, to see where the shoe pinches: they have committed themselves beforehand, and been talking what they know but little about. If I have, myself, taken some hundreds of the shower bath, and prescribed it to hundreds of others (as I have), I ought to know more concerning its effects

than those who have seldom or never attempted its use.
I do not say that a shower bath is the best that can be,
but I contend, that, properly managed, it is a most excellent mode. The pouring of water, or the small
stream, of the same quantity and force of the shower, I
hold is, in most cases, the best. I go, as I always have
done, for *avoiding* the shock, although this is generally
advocated as being the principal good of the bath. The
pouring, and the small stream, much less than the shower, produce a shock.

The rubbing sheet, affusions, sponging, hand or towel
washing, and the like means, are, as a rule, better in
pregnancy than the shower bath. Those, however,
who have suitable conveniencies, and can bear the
shower, may use it.

DOUCHE BATH.

The douche is a stream of water an inch, more or
less, in diameter, falling from a certain height. It may
be vertical, oblique, horizontal, or descending. That
which is nearly vertical is the one most used, and may
be considered as the only one strictly necessary in the
treatment, to produce the different effects required.
The ascending douche is, however, an excellent mode,
in cases of piles, and diseases of the uterine organs. As
a local means in uterine hæmorrhages, fluor albus, etc.,
this remedy is strikingly serviceable.

In the older works on water, we find the douche recommended, in various cases, to be taken upon the head.
This is, in every sense, wrong. The principal effect of
the douche, it is true, is the conduction of caloric from
the part upon which it is directed; still, the mechanical
force of the application is a sufficient objection against

its use upon that sensitive part, the head. The pouring, or affusion, upon this part, is always to be preferred. No blow of any kind should ever be struck upon the head.

Those who have weak lungs, stomach, or abdominal organs, should not take the douche upon those parts. Operate upon the system through the limbs, the large joints, and the muscular parts. This is the better mode. Weak organs can be strengthened, for most part, only through the general health.

In paralysis, and in diseased joints, the douche is a valuable remedy. In all cases of the like kinds, the system should be gradually prepared, by a general treatment. Persons are apt, here, as elsewhere, to have too great regard for local means, and not enough for general treatment. In diseases, of whatever kind, the greater part of the effect is to be brought about through the general means.

In gout and rheumatism, affecting the joints, there has been not a little discussion among medical writers, as to the safety of douching. It has been feared that the disease might be driven to some other part. Experience abundantly demonstrates, that of this there is not the slightest danger, provided certain plain rules are observed. If the part be hotter than is natural, so long is the application of cold water, by whatever means made, entirely safe. Indeed, we have no proof that cold water, in any case, ever produces the metastasis, or change of disease from one part to another, alluded to. If the part is not hotter than natural, the disease might become increased by the douche, but further than this, there is at least room for much doubt. The principal effect of cold external applications, it should be remembered, is the abstraction of heat. The action, then, is outward, and not inward, as is by some supposed. Another proof of this is the fact, that eruptions, boils, etc., appear upon the surface, where the water is used.

In some cases of swelled and painful joints, the relief obtained, in a very short time, by the douche, is little less than miraculous.

Old tumors are sometimes, in connection with other treatment, driven away in a very remarkable manner, by the action of the douche.

The best time for douching, I believe, in most cases, to be the morning. The system is then more vigorous from the night's rest, the stomach is more apt to be free from undigested food, and thus the strong impression of this powerful mode is the better borne. A strong douche should seldom be taken more than once a day.

A small douche is not so severe a bath as the shower. It does not abstract the heat so rapidly from the general system. But strong douching is not allowable in pregnancy.

THE HALF BATH.

This bath may be used as one of the mildest of water-cure processes, or as one of the most powerful. An ordinary bathing tub is a very good apparatus for the purpose. A good-sized washing tub will answer very well, if there is nothing else at hand. The water is generally quite shallow in this bath—from three to six inches. Priessnitz's half baths are made of wood, four to five feet long, about two and a half feet wide, and twenty inches deep. This simple contrivance is one of his most powerful means—that by which some of his highest triumphs are achieved. The water is generally used of moderate temperature, as 60 to 70 degrees Fah., and when long continued is changed, as it becomes warm from the heat of the body. This bath may be used—

1st. As a means of cooling the mass of the circulation in the hot stages of fevers, and inflammatory attacks of every kind.

2d. As a revulsive or means of deriving blood in congestions or inflammations of the larger organs, the brain, lungs, stomach, liver, etc.

3d. As a means of resuscitation in the shock of serious accidents, sun-stroke, and before, during, or after apoplectic and other fits. In drunkenness and delirium tremens, the half bath is a sovereign remedy.

4th. As a milder means, and preparatory to the general bath in weak constitutions.

In the latter of these indications the bath is generally used but for a few minutes, after the wet sheet, or at other times, as may be desired.

In the former indications, much practical knowledge is necessary in order to proceed always with safety and to obtain the best results. Thus six or even nine hours may be required, with the greatest perseverance, the patient being thoroughly rubbed over the whole surface, and this to be kept up constantly by relays of assistants, the patient's head and shoulders being supported meanwhile.

To make this bath milder for a given length of time, and more powerfully derivative downward, the upper half of the body is left warmly dressed, the frictions being carried on briskly upon the uncovered parts.

This bath is an excellent means in the paroxysms of ague and fever.

HEAD BATH.

From time immemorial, cooling applications to the head have been much depended upon in that violent and dangerous disease, phrenitis or inflammation of the brain. When all other means had failed, certain obstinate affections of the head have been known to give way by a constant stream or affusion of cold water upon the part. In headaches, convulsions, delirium tremens the delirium of fever, in epilepsy, rheumatism of the head, diseases of the eyes, earache, deafness, loss of smell and taste, and in epistaxis, or nose bleed, this highly energetic remedy is brought to bear.

In taking the head bath, the person lies at length upon a rug or matress, with perhaps a pillow under the shoulders. A broad, shallow basin or bowl of some kind is used. The back and sides of the head are in succession placed in the water. It may be taken for five minutes to a half hour, or even more, according to he case. The whole head should be well rubbed and dried, if there is no inflammation to combat.

Those who are under the necessity of going to excess in literary labors, or have much mental effort to put forth, will find great benefit from affusions upon the head and the head bath. Not unfrequently a troublesome headache will at once give way, by merely washing with cold water the part in which the pain exists.

In cases of inflammation of the brain, the patient should lay with his head extending a little way from the edge of the bed, and the head and shoulders supported by assistants, so that affusion of the coldest water may be kept up for hours if need be, a tub or other vessel being underneath to receive the water, the patient being at the same time in the wet sheet. I believe the affusion of ice-water can thus be better managed than any applications of ice in bladders and the like. Until not only the fever in the head, but that in the whole system is thoroughly reduced, this application cannot be overdone.

THE NASAL BATH.

In catarrh, colds in the head, and in diseases of the nasal passages, the sniffling of water up the nostrils is to be performed. The water should be drawn back and ejected by the mouth to obtain the best effects. This is a little disagreeable at first, but one soon becomes accustomed to it. In nose bleed this bath is a famous remedy ; for this purpose the colder the water the better.

Those who have injured the nasal cavities by snuff-taking, will find good to result from this bath. Some who have broken off the practice of snuff, use water instead, whenever they feel the want of the abominable thing.

THE MOUTH OR ORAL BATH.

For inflammations in the gums, mouth, throat, and palate, in slimy secretions from the throat, stomach, in toothache, catarrh, colds, and chronic hoarseness, garglings and baths for the mouth are of great service. Pauley, a merchant of Vienna, has been thought singular for his zeal in recommending this bath. Clergymen and others who suffer hoarseness by much speaking, will find that holding very cold water in the mouth until it begins to grow warm, and then ejecting it and by frequently repeating the process, much benefit will be obtained. Falling or elongation of the palate, in which

4

it is now so much of a professional hobby to clip off the part, the gargling sufficiently with cold water will be found a never-failing remedy. Coughs and tightness in the chest may often be essentially relieved by this bath. In mucous secretions from the throat and stomach, by ejecting the water a number of times, it will surprise those who have not witnessed the remedy, to see the amount of slimy secretion thrown off.

THE SITZ OR HIP BATH.

Convenient tubs, wooden or metallic, are constructed for this bath ; but an ordinary wash-tub answers very well. The article should be large enough to admit the motion of the arms in rubbing the abdomen, sides, and hips, first with one hand and then the other. Water enough is used generally to come pretty well up the abdomen. The more movement and friction, while in this bath, the better. It is more convenient if the tub be elevated two or three inches from the floor. Some undress completely and place a blanket or sheet over the upper part of the body, but oftener the parts only of the person to be exposed to the water are uncovered. In a variety of ailments, this bath is highly valuable. It may be made one of the most powerful of all of the hydropathic modes. Like all powerful applications, it should be made only after digestion is nearly or quite gone through with.

As a tonic to the stomach, liver, bowels, womb, spine, etc., this bath is highly useful. In constipation and other irregularities, it is famous. Those of sedentary habits will find its use of rare service. For the tonic effect, it is taken ten to twenty or twenty-five minutes or more. If it is continued some length of time, the water is to be changed once or more, as it would otherwise become too warm.

In pregnancy, besides general ablutions, the semi-daily use of this bath is productive of great good. In those troublesome itchings (*pruritus pudendi*), this application should be made as often as the symptoms occur, and the remedy will be found a sovereign one.

In all violent diseases of the abdominal organs, in which the parts are hotter than is natural, this bath is indicated. Prudence would here, as in all other modes, indicate that the cooling process be made not too sudden or long continued ; and one admirable feature of the system is, that experiments may be so safely made. The water may at first be made very moderate, so that a child can bear it ; and then, little by little, the temperature may be lowered without the least danger.

In severe inflammations of the chest or head, the cold hip bath is a powerful derivative, as we say in medicine. The excess of blood is thus drawn from the inflamed part, or parts, and the mass of the circulation cooled, and thus the pyrexia, or general feverishness, which is always present in inflammation, is removed.

In piles and hæmorrhoids, the cold hip bath is used, and in all acute diseases of the genital organs.

In that very common complaint, leucorrhœa, or the whites, this bath is very useful. There is also another admirable contrivance that may be used in connection— a small tube, or speculum, made of wire-work. It is about four inches long, and from half an inch to an inch, or more, in diameter. This, when introduced, allows the water to come in contact with the walls of the parts affected. These may be obtained at a trifling expense.

In violent flooding, the cold hip bath is a most powerful means. It should be undertaken only by those of experience in such cases.

In all violent bleedings from the bowels, very cold hip baths should be used. Let it be remembered, in all hæmorrhages, the parts at and about which the bleeding takes place are hotter than is natural, and that the constringing power of cold is the best possible means that can be resorted to. This is in accordance with all authority in the healing art.

Those most severe and troublesome itchings that sometimes torment pregnant females so much, and to the utter defiance of all ordinary remedies, are powerfully manageable by the hip bath.

THE COLD FOOT BATH.

The assertion put forth in some of the works on watercure, that the cold foot bath is to be prescribed for the same purpose that physicians order the warm, is, as I shall show, not true. The latter is prescribed among other remedies for the feet when cold. The former is not, as people have often been led to suppose, to be used while these parts are chilly. Some persons have, for instance, on going to bed, taken the cold foot bath, expecting the feet to become warmer, when to their surprise they find them only the colder, and that the parts remained in that condition for a longer time. So little do people observe and reason for themselves about some of the most common and simple things of life.

The feet, then, are first to be warm whenever the cold foot bath is taken. For various purposes, it is a most admirable remedy. For a tendency to cold feet, a very common symptom in these days of so-called luxury and ease, and one that indicates a state of things in the general system, incomparably more to be dreaded than the mere coldness of feet, this is *the* remedy. It may be taken at any convenient time. Just before the morning walk is very proper. The feet are then warm ; at other times, if cold, they should, if at all practicable, be warmed by exercise or frictions ; if this is not practicable, as in case of old age, debility, etc., the warm foot bath may, with advantage, be resorted to. The cold foot bath, in this case, should be shallow, covering only a part of the feet, and the water should be changed as it begins to grow lukewarm. Exercise, or at least friction, should be practiced after, as well as before the bath. The accustoming the feet thus to the impression of cold from day to day, will soon beget in them the condition of remaining habitually warm. The bath may be continued each time from a half to two or three hours, if desirable.

For toothache, rushing of blood to the head, ear and headache, inflamed eyes, etc., this bath is very useful. Also for controlling bleedings from the nostrils, the womb, and for difficulty in passing urine.

In cases of sprains of the feet and ancles, this bath, properly used, is a remedy of great power. In these cases, it should be at least deep enough to cover the parts affected. Pregnant women will find great relief in hot weather, by often washing the feet.

THE PEDILUVIUM, OR WARM FOOT BATH.

The warm foot bath, the " soaking the feet," of the days of our good sires and grandames of old, is, in its place, a most excellent part of " water-cure." It is used

4*

for soothing pains and aches that are of a nervous character, and for sometimes warming the feet when cold. It is often pleasanter, and by far better to warm the feet well in the warm foot bath on going to bed, rather than to remain an hour or more awake for the want of warm feet. Then, as we have said, in the morning when the feet are warm, take the cold foot bath. This will, so to speak, get those parts in the habit of becoming warm.

GENERAL DIRECTIONS CONCERNING BATHS.

Persons who are under the necessity of commencing the use of water, without the advice of a physician (and most persons in chronic disease, with the most perfect safety, may), should begin very cautiously. It is so easy, at any time, to increase, that there is no need of hurry in the matter. "Haste makes waste." Begin by merely washing the surface once, daily. If you are very weak and sensitive, use the water at 70 degrees Fah., or even 80 degrees, and if it is at 90 degrees, it is yet cooling,—cold water, in effect, and very mild in degree. It is easy, then, to lower the temperature, day by day, as you find you can bear. Rub the skin thoroughly, to excite activity in this part. The warmer it becomes, and the better the circulation, the more grateful is water, and the better the effect accomplished. Very soon you can commence taking the shower, small stream, or douche, upon a part. Take it first upon a single limb or two, next upon all the limbs, then upon a part of the body, and finally upon the whole, except the head. In this way, any one, who is able to walk about, may gradually and safely accustom himself to the shower, or small douche bath. Most persons are apt to wish to proceed too rapidly, and, in so doing, fail of bringing about the best results. If disease has been a long time accumulating, as is almost always true, time must be given for Nature to do her work. You may aid her in her efforts, but to force her is impossible. Many invalids, of course, have strength to proceed much more rapidly than I have indicated for those who are very weak. But, I repeat, those who practice upon themselves, should proceed cautiously, and, as it were, feel their way.

If one bath per day is found useful, soon a second may be ventured upon, and finally a third, or even a fourth. Weak persons go fishing voyages, and, in many cases, soon become able to remain much in the water, the whole day, and half of the night. If a crisis appears, you may know Nature is doing her work. The treatment must then be moderated somewhat for a time.

HOW OFTEN SHOULD WE BATHE?

There appears to be as good reason for the daily cleansing of the whole surface as of the hands and face. I have before written, "Every sick person, in whatever condition, or however weak, should have the whole body rubbed over, with wet cloths, sponges, etc., at least once each day. In some cases, great caution will be required, in order that the bath be performed safely. Let those who have lain for days upon a sick bed, without any ablution, as is generally the case in the ordinary modes of medical practice, try, when the body is warm the rubbing it part by part over the whole surface, following, briskly, with dry cloths, and then covering it warmly according to the feelings of comfort, and they will find it a most effectual tonic, as well as an application productive of the greatest comfort. Physicians generally have yet many simple lessons of this kind to learn."

Let every individual, then, old and young, male and female, sick or well, have a daily bath: and in case of indisposition, of whatever kind, let there be more, instead of less, than usual attention given to bathing.

Especially let pregnant women observe daily ablutions. In no condition of the system is water more safe and salutary than in this.

CHAPTER III.

COMPRESSES OR BANDAGES, AND THE WET SHEET.

Wet Compresses or Bandages Important Means of Water-Cure.—Cooling Compresses.—The Warming or Stimulating.—The Soothing.—Warm and Hot Fomentations.—The Wet Girdle.—Its Mode of Application and Uses.—Oil and India Rubber Cloth Bandages.—The German Water Dressing for Wounds, Cuts, etc.—The Wet Sheet.—Mode of Applying it.—Its Soothing Effects.—Not to be Used for Sweating.—Bathing after the Sheet.—Wet Sheets in Fevers and Inflammations.—Becoming Cold in the Wet Sheet.—Heat and Fullness in the Head —The Wet Sheet applicable in Pregnancy.

COMPRESSES OR BANDAGES.

WET compresses or bandages are important applications in the water-cure. They perform precisely the same office upon a *part* of the system, as the wet sheet upon the *whole* system.

Cooling Wet Compresses are such as are changed or re-wet frequently, until the necessary amount of coolness is obtained. These are applicable to any part.

Warming, or Stimulating Wet Compresses, are, in their secondary effects, the opposite of the cooling. Covered, and left upon the part a sufficient length of time, the surface becomes warm, and even warmer than is natural, in consequence of the retained heat. They are therefore said to be *warming,* or *stimulating.*

A distinction may be made between the cooling and the warming. Such as give no decided sensation of either coolness or warmth, may be said to be soothing in effect.

There are certain pains, as of the spasmodic kind, in which I believe hot applications are best. In some forms of pleurisy, colic, and in other deep-seated internal pains, I should, in my own case, were I attacked, resort first to very hot applications in order to lull the pain. I would, at the same time, use cooling means for the general system, as circumstances should require. Years ago, I took a deep-seated inflammation in the region of the kidneys. I reduced the pains, which were at times very severe, quickly and effectually, simply by having placed at the small of the back, hot bricks wrapped in wet cloths. The remedy acted like a charm, did not weaken my system, but, on the contrary, indirectly made me strong. When the pain was on, I was in the greatest distress, and could not, without the greatest difficulty, walk, stand, or sit. When it was off again, I could run, jump, and do any thing I pleased. I was a part of the time where nothing could be done; but in every instance, when I could have the bricks, I at once drove off the pain, and was very soon cured. We all know that heat, as a general fact, is weakening; so also is cold, if used to excess. We should always use as little of artifical warmth as may be, but if we can relieve pain without debilitating the general system, we do well.

Hot and warm fomentations have, in some form or other, been long resorted to in the healing art. The French, more particularly, have for many years adopted this simple remedy. The principal part of medical treatment in France, is that called the expectant—the watching mode, as it may be called. Medicines are not depended upon for specific effects. Almost no medicine is given. Cooling or warming and diluting drinks, topical applications, injections, etc., together with great care in diet, are among the principal means. In fevers, and in cases attended with visceral irritation, i. e., slight inflammation or uneasiness of the internal organs, the warm or hot fomentation is much used.

Dr. Gully, of England, very strongly advocates this remedy, and, in following the French, gives the following directions for its use: "A piece of flannel, thrice folded, is placed into a dry basin, and very hot or warm water is poured on it, sufficiently to soak it. The flannel is then put into the corner of a towel, which is twisted round it and wrung until the flannel is only damp. It is taken out of the towel, and immediately placed over the part to be fomented, and upon it is placed a double fold of thick flannel, dry, or a part of a light blanket. The patient, then, if it be the abdomen which is fomented, draws the ordinary bed-clothes over him, and remains quiet five or eight minutes, when another flannel, freshly wrung out, is applied, the former one being withdrawn. And this goes on for the whole time prescribed for the fomentation."

Dr. Gully praises this application in the strongest terms; thus he observes: "Often and again I have seen it procure sleep to adults, and to children especially, when opiates only fevered and irritated. I have seen it, applied at night, procure relaxation of the kidneys and bowels by the morning, when all diuretics and purgatives had failed. I have seen it arrest the most violent bilious and nervous headaches. I have seen it stay fits of the asthma, of tic douloureux of the face, of toothache, of sciatica (hip disease), of spasms of the bladder, of universal convulsions in infants, both from teething and indigestion. I have seen it stop the most violent and long-continued vomiting, and relieve, even during the application, extreme acidity and flatulence of the stomach."

We should remember things we all know now to be injurious, have been as strongly recommended as this. At the same time, be it observed, warm water does not poison, irritate, or inflame the system. The application is made only to a part of the surface. Pains and uneasiness are removed, and the patient at once gains much in comfort and in strength.

THE WET GIRDLE.

This application, which all hydropathists so much esteem, is more or less used in almost every case. Patients should generally wear it, at least, a part of the day. Three yards of strong toweling make a good and convenient girdle. If a person is very sensitive, a half-yard only, enough of one end to cover the front of the body, is wet. It is girded just above the hips, and drawn quite tight about the lower part of the abdomen; but at the upper part, it should be left loose enough for breathing easily. In cold weather, those who are very sensitive, and cannot exercise enough to keep warm, may use only one or two yards about the body, covered with flannel to secure warmth. People are too apt to fear cold, and should practice themselves always to bear as much as they can. Some wear the girdle night and day. It should be wet every few hours, at most, and not be allowed to get dry, although there is no danger in that. It is best, I believe, to wear it not all of the twenty-four hours. Some have it by night, when business does not admit of it during the day. If arranged by the person's self, it should first, after being wet, be rolled like a scroll, as surgeons' bandages are, and thus it may be readily applied.

If one is sensitive and weak, and the girdle is too heavy, too much wet, or the person too inactive, some form of a cold may then be brought on but this does not often take place. If too much covering is used, or the girdle not sufficiently wet, or is too light in texture, too much heat may then be retained. The body becomes feverish, and some injury is done. If every thing is properly arranged, it has a powerfully strengthening effect, as those who have adopted its use well know.

The wet girdle is of great service in pregnancy. If properly used, it aids much in keeping up the general strength, and in procuring good sleep, upon which so much depends. Do not let it become too warm.

OIL AND INDIA RUBBER CLOTH BANDAGES

Should never be worn over the wet cloths. Evaporation should be allowed, so that effete and morbid matters may be driven off. These coverings protect the clothing from moisture, which is sometimes a convenience, but, as a rule, they should not be allowed.

Many of the first surgeons and physicians of Europe have recommended the German water dressing, as it is called, in preference to any other. I am not entirely certain, but have no doubt that Priessnitz has been the principal means of this improvement. Dr. Billing, of London, one of the first and most experienced physicians of the day, in a late work, says: "The German water dressing has much the advantage over the poultice; the piece of lint dipped in water is lighter than the

5

poultice; the oiled silk over all retains the moisture, and the whole does not spoil the sound skin, as the poultice often does.   If poultices be too long applied, proud flesh will form, either from a superfluous growth of healthy granulations, or of such as are weak or spongy." Professor Mütter, of Philadelphia, in notes to a recent work of Professor Liston, one of the first surgeons of Europe, agrees with the latter in the superiority of the water dressing in wounds and injuries.   "In lacerated wounds, to which Mr. Liston refers in the text," says Dr. M., "no dressing is comparable to water, in some form or other, and for several years I have employed as a first dressing, nothing else.   In summer, I use cold, and in winter, warm, and apply it as recommended by Liston and McCartney, viz.: after cleansing the wound and approximating its edges, whenever this is proper, pledgets of patent lint, dipped in water, are to be gently laid upon its surface, and the whole covered with a piece of oiled silk (flannel is quite sufficient), to prevent evaporation.   In summer I have found it best not to apply the oiled silk, as it keeps the part too hot, and in its stead apply two thicknesses of wet lint, which will retain the moisture much longer than one.   An assistant should also, about every half hour, pour a spoonful of water over the dressings, but without removing them. Thus treated, I have seen the most terrific lacerated wounds from machinery or gun-shot, heal most rapidly by the first intention.   Only a few weeks since, I treated the son of a professional friend, who had received a severe lacerated wound, with the loss of a portion of two fingers, from the bursting of his gun, by the cold water dressing, and nearly every fragment of skin that could be placed in a proper position, united by the first intention." Water, to promote animal growth in any part, is as serviceable as in the vegetable productions of the earth. I have said elsewhere, that it is through the medium of water all vital processes, whether animal or vegetable, are carried on. It is not strange that the virtues of water to *heal*, incomparably the best of all substances, were not, until of late, becoming generally known, since there is in the human mind such a tendency to the marvelous and mystical.

THE WET SHEET.

The usual mode of applying the wet sheet, is thus : a number of woollen blankets are spread evenly upon a bed or matress ; a sheet, of cotton or linen material (linen is the more cooling), is spread smoothly upon the blankets ; the patient then lays at length upon the sheet. This is lapped over from side to side, and made to cover the whole surface ; the blankets, one by one, are in like manner adjusted, drawn tightly, and well tucked under each side. Large pins or tapes may be used, to secure these coverings. The blankets should be well arranged about the neck and feet, to prevent evaporation and too great chilliness. A down or feather bed is sometimes put over the whole, and tucked under, the more effectually to retain the warmth. If there is a tendency to coldness of the feet, these may be left covered with the blankets only. Faithful rubbing them with the hand is a good mode. Working and rubbing them one against the other is serviceable ; and rather than allow these parts to remain a long time cold, as is sometimes done, it would be better to place moderately warm bricks, or, better, bottles of warm water, etc., to them ; and the same may be said of any part of the system. Some fear warm applications in water-cure, seeming to believe that every thing must be of a cold, chilling kind. The fact is, *warm* applications, though seldom needed, are, under certain conditions, as natural, as scientific, as the *cold*, under other conditions. Still, it is always better, as far as possible, to cause the body to create its own warmth.

The first reclining upon the cold sheet is, of course, unpleasant; but, every thing properly arranged, a most soothing sensation begins soon to pervade the system, and it is no exaggeration to say, that if a person's state of bodily or mental health had been such that he had determined upon suicide, he would soon change his mind in the matter.

The sensations caused by the wet sheet are so delicious, persons are very apt to remain in it too long. As a general fact, it will be found best to remain in it only long enough to become tolerably warm. Many have an idea that *sweating* should always take place, and some *practitioners* have been in the habit of sweating their patients into a nightmare. They seem to imagine that sweating is the one great thing to be sought. This is wrong, and, once for all, it should be understood, *that sweating is of itself a debilitating process.* The times for it are the exceptions, and not the rule. Priessnitz does not, latterly, allow any one to remain in the sheet over twenty minutes at a time, without coming out of it, or at least changing the sheet.

Some form of bath should be given after the wet sheet, not that it is absolutely required in all instances to be safe, but, on the whole, it is more beneficial so to do. The surface now needs cleansing, and the invigorating effect of cold water. If a person is weak, and not able to sit up, the water should be used tepid, as at 70 or 75 degrees Fah. Piecemeal, with wet towels, the body is to be rubbed, until dry; and it is better to obtain a comfortable glow. A half bath may be taken, or a shower, plunge, or spout bath, as the case may be. As in all other applications, those who have not the advice of an experienced physician, should begin with the milder modes, and then proceed gradually to the stronger, as they ascertain, by experiment, what they can bear.

In diseases attended with an increase of heat of the general system, the cooling wet sheet is indicated. There is no danger here, so long as the animal heat is above the natural standard. If it be high, burning fever use two or three sheets at a time, and thus the refrigerant action will be longer continued. Little covering, other than the sheets, need be used, in cases of high fever, and sometimes none at all. If the body is becoming cooled too fast, and shiverings occur, more covering is then applied. The sheets should be changed as often as they become too warm, and as many times as is necessary to reduce the fever, be it three or fifty times in the day. Half baths, ablutions, affusions, etc., will be serviceable between times. If the system should at any time become too much chilled, the warming means are to be resorted to, packing in warm blankets, warm baths, and the like.

Some persons, who seem not to have much calorific power, are at first, that is, after a few minutes, comfortable, but, in twenty or thirty minutes, feel chilly, although to another their body appears not so. Persons in such cases should come from the sheet while

5*

yet feeling warm.   Should it be desirable to continue
longer, the rubbing wet-sheet first, and then the dry,
may be applied briskly, to excite circulation and warmth.
The wet sheet envelopment may then a second time be
used.   The better way, however, is to take the second
sheet a half hour or so at another time of the day.   A
half hour in the early part of the day, and another in
the after part, is worth much more than the two in succession.

This tendency to after-chilliness in the sheet is soon
driven off, if every thing is managed in such way that
the patient gradually gains strength.

The wet sheet, used with moderation, is an excellent
means in pregnancy.   Used with proper caution, no one
need be afraid of it.

CHAPTER IV.

DISORDERS OF PREGNANCY.

Febrile Condition of the System during the period of Pregnancy.—This may be great-ly Modified by Diet, and general Regimen.—Protecting Power of Pregnancy.—Dis-eased Persons should not Procreate.—Acute Diseases more dangerous in Preg-nancy.—Harsh Means not allowable during this Period.—Insomnia or Sleeplessness in Pregnancy.—How to be Prevented.—Headache.—Sometimes a dangerous Symptom in Pregnancy.—The Remedial Means.—Sick or Nervous Headache.—Tea and Coffee often Causes of this Disease.—Breeding with a Toothache.—How to be Remedied.—Teeth not to be Extracted during Pregnancy.—Salivation.—This is often a Troublesome Complaint.—How it is to be Remedied.—Difficulty in Breath-ing.—Heart-Burn.—Too much Food generally a Cause.—Means of Preventing it.

FEBRILE CONDITION OF THE SYSTEM DURING THE PERIOD OF PREGNANCY.

PREGNANCY is always attended with more or less ex-citement of the system, an excitement which bears some resemblance to a state of fever. There is also a greater proneness to fevers, even from slight causes, now than at other times. Hence the necessity of avoiding, as far as possible, all such causes; and hence also, the neces-sity of exercising the greatest care, in regard to diet and drinks. Too much food, and that which is too exciting, will cause more harm in pregnancy than at other times, from the greater tendency to fever. The common be-lief among women is, that more food is needed during pregnancy than at other times, because the food goes to furnish nourishment for two instead of one, that is, for the mother and the child within her. "It is therefore,"

says Dr. Dewees, "constantly recommended to eat and
drink heartily ; and this she too often does, until the system is goaded to fever ; and sometimes to more sudden
and greater evils, as convulsions or apoplexy."

If, instead of full diet, women in pregnancy will but
try the plan of eating less food, even of becoming very
abstemious, they will most assuredly find that they get
along better, suffer less from plethora or fullness, and
enjoy greater comfort of body in every respect.

There is a mechanical reason—one which females
themselves can best understand—why less food should
be taken during pregnancy than at other times ; the abdomen is more full at this period ; much more so
toward the end of pregnancy.   Hence it is that at this
time a full meal will cause a greater sense of fullness,
and in every respect a greater degree of discomfort,
than when pregnancy does not exist.

PROTECTING POWER OF PREGNANCY.

It is generally regarded that pregnancy exerts a protecting influence against many diseases, particularly
those of epidemic kind.   This is probably not always
true.   The very reverse of this rule is said to have occurred in some instances of prevailing disease.   Consumption, that dread *American* disease, appears usually
to be arrested, for the time being, in its career by pregnancy.   But sad is the state of the sufferer after the
period has closed.   What the disease had lost in time
by the pregnancy, it now makes up in violence and fearful speed.   It is a sad thing for a really consumptive
woman to become pregnant—sad for herself and not
less so for her offspring.   Think of a child being formed

out of the blood and fluids of a mother whose system is already in a deeply diseased and almost corrupt state. It were a miracle almost if such a child could, by any possibility, ever enjoy health. It is a wrong thing for diseased parents to beget their kind.

ACUTE DISEASES, AS AFFECTED BY PREGNANCY.

It is said to have been an aphorism of Hippocrates, the father of medicine, who lived more than two thousand years ago, that pregnant women attacked with acute disease always die. This strong assertion cannot be said to hold good, certainly at the present day; but yet pregnancy, it must be admitted, exercises, as a general fact, a very unfavorable influence on the system in acute disease. The danger here may be said to be three-fold. First, the system is already in a febrile condition, or one very nearly bordering thereon; second, there is the new disease; and third, this often causes the death of the fœtus (unborn child), and then the dangers of abortion are superadded upon the others. "The life of the child, too," say authors, "is endangered by the treatment necessary for the cure; especially in the use of harsh purgatives, violent emetics, salivation, and profuse bleedings." But thanks to a better day, we of the water practice are under no necessity of running such fearful risks. We have not only a more effectual way, but one, when managed by judicious hands, harmless and safe. "It is by the prompt use of mild means, and a persevering attention to small matters," judiciously observes Dr. Maunsel, "that the patient is to be conducted through the dangers that encompass her." And he justly adds, "Above all, avoid the dreadful blunder of treating a woman for acute disease without discovering that she is pregnant."

INSOMNIA, OR WANT OF SLEEP.

Sleeplessness, to a greater or less degree, not unfrequently occurs during pregnancy. This is most apt to occur during the later months of pregnancy. Within a few days of the birth, however, better rest is experienced, and a greater degree of comfort in every respect. This tendency to sleeplessness during pregnancy is sometimes so troublesome as almost wholly to prevent sleep. "The limbs are agitated by involuntary contractions of the muscles, which by the frequency and suddenness of their motion, instantly interrupt the sleep to which the woman was at the moment strongly inclined."

"Sleeplessness," says Dr. Maunsel, "most frequently affects the weak, nervous, and irritable, occurring sometimes early in pregnancy, oftener toward the end of the term. If the want of sleep continue for many days, it is commonly followed by very grave symptoms, as restlessness, fever, mental disturbance, convulsions, etc.; abortion has resulted from it, and some cases have terminated in insanity; others have destroyed life." But those who follow a judicious course of the water-treatment do not become thus afflicted. If such occurrences should be at all possible in the new modes, the cases would be exceedingly rare. I have known many persons to follow bathing during pregnancy, but none who have had any thing like serious difficulty in obtaining sleep.

In many cases this want of sleep in pregnancy does not sensibly impair the general health. Some persons have been under the necessity of walking their room much of the night ; and yet after a short repose at the dawn of day, have been astonished to find themselves as much refreshed, apparently, as after a good night's rest.

To prevent sleeplessness in pregnancy a variety of means have been recommended. If there is plethora or too great fullness of the system, small bleedings and cooling purgatives of mild kind are recommended by almost every author who has written on the subject. It is well known that in many parts of the country, women believe that they cannot get through pregnancy at al without being bled. The doctors have been at the root of this matter in the beginning. This old-fashioned practice fortunately is now fast going out of date. It is not for me here to enter into a discussion of the question whether such means ever do any good in pregnancy ; but I will say, on the authority of physiological and pathological science, and my own experience, that bathing, water-drinking, and the proper regulation of the general habits, are incomparably the best modes ; the best, not only for the time of pregnancy, but also for that of childbirth and the period of nursing.

Dr. Dewees recommended for this affection, low diet, cool air, and cold water, as being among the best remedies. And Dr. Denman says, that " a glass of cold water drank at bed-time is not a contemptible remedy ;" and he might have said one of the best, especially if the dose be soon repeated. And Dr. Dewees, in quoting this advice of Dr. Denman, adds, " We know that bathing the hands and face in cold water is an excellent one, and should always be resorted to."

Dr. Maunsel says, " Pediluvia (foot baths), or what is better, hip baths, very often do good." But the important matter of temperature, the doctor does not speak of. A warm hip bath and a cold one are very different things. He remarks, also, well, "that the diet should be cooling, and exercise in the open air as freely as circumstances will permit."

I may, however, dismiss this whole matter of sleeplessness in pregnancy, by saying, that those who bathe daily, exercise judiciously, and, when possible, in the open air, drink only pure soft water (and all can have this from the clouds), partake only of plain and unstimulating food, and sleep upon hard beds and pillows, in cool fresh air, will rarely, if ever, be troubled with want of sleep.

One other thing, however; it sometimes seems necessary for persons in pregnancy to get a "nap" during the day. Those who have great cares, and many in our country have, often find it extremely difficult to get through the long, hot days of summer without sleep. Now, in such cases, if the woman can go by herself, and be wholly undisturbed, and feel entirely free from every care, and thus get a good half hour or an hour's sleep, she will be much refreshed thereby. It is necessary to observe that the clothing should be removed as at night. Persons often wonder how it is that they feel worse after sleeping than before. When one lies down, if the clothing be left on, too much heat is retained about the surface, and thus debility instead of refreshment is experienced. This day-sleeping should be done with the stomach empty, as at three or more hours after a meal, and not in the afternoon, as that would be liable to cause wakefulness at night. It is truly surprising how much, under favorable circumstances, a short sleep even will refresh the powers of life.

HEADACHE.

A headache in pregnancy—one which occurs often, and is not a sick or nervous headache—is regarded by authors generally as a very serious affair. It occurs mostly in the later months of the period, and is attended with plethora or general fullness of the system, throbbing at the temples, suffusion of the eyes, ringing in the ears, indistinct vision, and flashes of light passing before the eyes. If this headache gets to be very severe, *splitting*, as we may say, there is danger of either apoplexy or puerperal convulsions. But these things, be it remembered, do not come upon those who live moderately, exercise in the open air, and practice daily ablutions.

According to the old practice, prompt and decided means must be at once taken in such cases; not, however, so powerful as would be admissible when pregnancy does not exist.

Fasting, bathing, frequent yet moderate exercise in the open air, sleeping in large, cool, and well ventilated rooms, with frequent washings of the head in cold water, and cooling bandages upon the head, are by far better as well as safer means than bleeding and purgatives, usually resorted to on such occasions.

SICK OR NERVOUS HEADACHE.

Dr. Maunsel says of nervous headache in pregnancy, "This, especially if it take the form of hemicrania (pain confined to one half of the head), is one of the most unmanageable of the diseases of pregnancy." And of the remedies recommended, the doctor speaks as follows: "If the state of the system indicates bleeding, it will

6

commonly do good ; local should be preferred to general bleeding.   If this is not indicated, we should first
attend to the secretions; when these are corrected,
antispasmodics and anodynes come in well.   Hyoscia-
mus and camphor, a grain each, is a good remedy ; also
the volatile tincture of valereau.   The external application of some anodyne extract, as stramonium, belladona,
or cicata, may be tried, but with caution, lest they produce the poisonous effects of the drug."

Now compare with the above practice of bleeding
and dosing, *secundum artem*, the true and rational one
In nineteen cases out of twenty, the nervous headache
comes from either tea or coffee drinking, or the use of
improper food.   Only remove the causes then, and the
difficulty vanishes.   Strange to say, however, there are
many women who have either so little confidence in
what any one can say to them, or so little control over
themselves, they will not even make the experiment.
Should one who has been cured tell them the fact,
they will not yet believe ; nor would they if one should
rise from the dead.   Such persons, those who have the
truth set before them and yet will not act, are welcome
to all their tea and coffee, their fine food, their bleeding
and dosing, and their sick headache.

TOOTHACHE.

Breeding with a toothache is an old proverb.   Tooth
ache is certainly more apt to occur during pregnancy
than at other times, and not unfrequently it is a very
early symptom of this state.   And what may appear
singular, the teeth ache without being diseased.   Especially those who drink strong tea and coffee are more

subject to this nervous toothache, as we may term it; toothache where there is no decay. Ceasing with the cause, then, is the surest means of relief. It is dangerous to extract teeth in the early months of pregnancy. The operation has been often known to cause immediate abortion. There is the greater danger of this in the early months.

Bleeding has often been practiced for this affection in pregnancy; but that is a worse than useless resort, and moreover, generally fails of the object. After a few days of full diet, the affection is quite certain to return, and appears to be even the more obstinate for the bleeding. Fasting, with water-drinking, is a much better mode. Very seldom will toothache withstand twenty-four hours entire abstinence from all food. If the face has become much swelled, of course so great relief could not be experienced in so short a time. But even then the fasting is of incalculable good. General bathing, and going into the open air, are also excellent means. The rubbing sheet is particularly applicable. And Dr. Burns, in his work on Midwifery, years ago said, "Sometimes a little cold water held in the mouth, abates the pain." This will be the case whenever the toothache is one of inflammation; but if it be of the more nervous kind, warm water will give more relief. If the nerve is much exposed, it is perhaps always best to hold warm, or at least lukewarm water in the mouth, and at the same time to practice very brisk and continued rubbing of the face, temples, neck, etc., with the hand wet often in cold water. Wet bandages upon the face are also good. If the aching be of the nervous kind, that is, without inflammation, warm bandages often repeated afford the most relief.

SALIVATION.

There is often a greater or less degree of salivation during the period of pregnancy. Probably all women experience at this time, a more than ordinary flow of saliva. This sometimes becomes very excessive and troublesome to the patient, especially at night, when the sleep is disturbed by the frequent necessity of emptying the mouth. Dewees observes : " It is almost always accompanied with acidity of the stomach, and constipation of the bowels ; the fluid discharged from the mouth, for the most part, is perfectly colorless and transparent ; at other times, it is more tenacious and frothy, and the quantity poured out is sometimes incredibly profuse. It almost always has an unpleasant taste, though not attended with an offensive smell ; it keeps the stomach in a constant state of irritation, and not unfrequently provokes vomiting, especially if the saliva be tenacious, and requires an effort to discharge it." Dr. Dewees relates a case where this affection commenced at the second month of pregnancy, in which the patient discharged daily from one to three quarts of salivary fluid, and became so weakened thereby, that she was unable to sit up without immediately fainting.

The above description of salivation in pregnancy may be said to apply to patients who live according to the ordinary modes of society. I have, during six years past, known many women who have passed through pregnancy, practicing at the same time daily bathing, water-drinking exercising regularly in the open air, with plain diet, and in no instance have I known salivation to prove at all inconvenient or troublesome. I judge that this affection, if such we may call it, can only come on when the general health is at fault, or the dietetic and other hygienic habits bad. True, there is probably always more or less increase of the salivary secretions in pregnancy, but if good habits are daily persevered n, I think no one will be troubled at all in this matter.

DIFFICULTY OF BREATHING.

Toward the latter months of pregnancy, there is always, necessarily, more or less difficulty of breathing. The uterus becomes so large, and fills so much of the abdomen, that the upward and downward motion of the diaphragm, or partition between this and the chest, is greatly impeded. Hence the dyspnœa, or difficulty of breathing. A cough, likewise, not unfrequently attends this symptom, and becomes so severe in some cases as to cause abortion.

Great and protracted exertion, severe fatigue of whatever kind, bodily or mental, ought to be avoided during pregnancy. Running up stairs too quickly, walking too rapidly, and any undue mental excitement, increases this difficulty of breathing. Some mothers are in the habit of taking up heavy children needlessly and carrying them, which is one of the most certain means of doing harm to themselves. So also inaction is bad for the breathing. If the individual do not have exercise enough to answer the purposes of health, the system becomes more plethoric or full, and thus also the difficulty is increased. The medium of neither too little nor too much should always be observed. The same also may be said of the diet. And here I remark, that if any pregnant woman will carefully make the experiment, she will find that in the latter months of pregnancy, an **exceedingly**

6*

small allowance of food only, with free water-drinking bathing, and moderate exercise in the open air, will be sufficient to keep up her strength, and that in a most remarkable manner. Let her not be deluded by the old maxim, that because there are two to support she must take a greater amount of food.

HEART-BURN.

Heart-burn is not unfrequently one of the first unpleasant symptoms that women experience after becoming pregnant. This sometimes becomes very distressing, and difficult to manage according to the ordinary modes. "It is generally," says Dr. Dewees, "very distressing and very difficult to subdue." He had known large and repeated doses of the alkalies given with scarcely any temporary alleviation, and much less, permanent benefit.

The great cause of heart-burn in pregnancy as well as in other cases, is acidity of the stomach; and acidity of the stomach comes from improper food. Very seldom, indeed, can a pregnant woman be troubled with heart-burn, acidity of the stomach, or vomiting, if the dietetic and other habits be regulated according to principle. Pregnant women, in this country of abundance, generally eat a great deal too much food. They have also too little exercise in the open air. Some, indeed, have too much exercise, as in doing household work; but more are injured by doing too little than too much. But in this country ninety-nine of the one hundred *eat too much food while in the pregnant state.*

To cure the heart-burn, let the woman, when she first experiences it, at once desist in the quantity of food.

If she rises in the morning and finds the symptom upon her, she may be certain that digestion has gone on badly the day previous, and that the stomach contains portions of the undigested aliment which has passed into the acetous fermentation, and thus causing the difficulty she experiences. What is to be done in such a case? Will the introduction of another portion of food into the already disordered stomach make matters any the better? Certainly not, except for a short time. When the stomach is goaded on by a new meal, the individual may feel the better for half an hour; but, other things being equal, it in the end only makes the matter worse. Fasting a meal or two, with water-drinking for its tonic effect, is the best possible means. The stomach thus has time to regain its vigor, and food taken in moderation, subsequently, will then be found to agree perfectly well. It will here also surprise any one to learn how small an amount of food is really necessary, with water-drinking, to sustain the strength.

If the heart-burn is very troublesome, it will be found of great relief for the patient to vomit by means of water. This, in most cases, will take place very easily by drinking, in quick succession, a number of tumblers of soft water, about blood-warm temperature. This, with a little help, as by putting the finger in the throat, will be found sufficient; and if, in any case, the vomiting does not take place, the water yet does much good by means of diluting the offending matters in the stomach. Thus suppose there is one ounce of acid matters in the gastric cavity, and that ten ounces of pure water are introduced therein, the offending mass is weakened tenfold; so that even if vomiting does not take place, great relief is experienced. I would not have any one make too great an effort to produce vomiting, especially in pregnancy, for hard vomiting might cause abortion. There is, however, no danger except the vomiting caused by drug substances. Water-vomiting is easier than can be imagined by those who have tried only the old modes.

Soda and other alkalies, taken so often to ease heart-burn, do more harm than good in the end. The wet girdle, worn occasionally about the abdomen, and managed so as to produce a cooling effect, will be found of great service in invigorating the stomach, thus tending to prevent heart-burn, acidity, and the like. So also the general ablutions, which ought never, for a single day, to be omitted during pregnancy, as we may say too of other times.

In heart-burn, arising from whatever cause, it is a very common custom, both with the profession and the people, to give alkalies, as magnesia and chalk. Dr. Dewees tells us that he had known large and repeated doses given, with scarcely any temporary alleviation, much less permanent benefit. It is of little effect, certainly, to continue giving these articles, when at the same time the dietetic habits are such as are certain of keeping up the difficulty. This would hold true even if the articles administered were perfectly neutral in their effects as to harm, which can never be the case. All drug substances, however much good they do, at the same time cause a certain amount of harm. The articles, magnesia and chalk, the ones generally resorted to in this difficulty, are moreover often impure. This is particularly true of chalk.

Dr. Dewees mentions a case in which the lady's health was utterly destroyed by her enormous use of chalk. "I formerly attended a lady, with several children," says he, "who was in the habit of eating chalk during the whole term of pregnancy; she used it in such excessive quantities as to render the bowels almost useless. I have often known her without an evacuation for ten or twelve days together, and then it was only procured by enemata (injections); and the dejections were literally chalk. Her calculation, I well remember, was three half-pecks for each pregnancy; she became as white nearly as the substance itself; and it eventually destroyed her, by so deranging her stomach that it would retain nothing upon it."

CHAPTER V.

DISORDERS OF PREGNANCY—(*Continued*)

Nausea and Vomiting.—These Symptoms more common in the early months of Pregnancy.—What Persons are most subject to them.—Vomiting sometimes becomes Dangerous.—How Nausea and Vomiting are to be Prevented.—Morbid Craving or Longing for particular articles of food in Pregnancy.—These should not be gratified.—Pain in the Right Side.—How to be Remedied.—Constipation.—This is most common in the earlier months of Gestation.—Causes of Constipation.—Remedial Means to be Used.—These the same as in Constipation ordinarily.—Diarrhœa in Pregnancy.—Not so frequent as Constipation.—Both to be treated on the same General Principles.—Piles and Hæmorrhoids.—Modes of Treatment.—Difficulty of voiding Urine.—How to be Remedied.—Itching of the Genital Parts.—Water a sovereign Remedy.—Swelling of the Limbs.—Varicose Veins.—Cramps in the Lower Extremities.—Pain in the Breasts.—How to be treated.—Warm or hot Applications sometimes Useful.—The Mind as affected by Pregnancy.—Women are more apt to become irritable at this time.—Hysteria in Pregnancy.

NAUSEA AND VOMITING.

Nausea and vomiting are frequent occurrences during the early months of pregnancy. Various conjectures have been put forth concerning the causes of these symptoms, one of which is, that they act in preventing plethora, or too great fullness of the system. But it may be asked, if this is so, why do they not continue in the later months of gestation, when plethora is still more prejudicial than in the early months? The plain truth in the matter appears to be this: those persons who are feeble and have depraved health—those who sleep upon feather beds, who are inactive in their habits, who drink tea and coffee, and subsist on fine and concentrated food, such as is almost certain to cause indigestion, and to keep up a state of constipated bowels—are by far the most apt to suffer from nausea and vomiting in pregnancy. Those who have good constitutions, and live consistently in all respects—practicing daily bathing, water-drinking, etc.—are troubled but very little with these symptoms.

These suggestions, then, indicate the modes of cure for this complaint. Reform *all* the habits. If this does not effect the object, there need be no fears entertained. If the food is then rejected by the stomach, we may infer that the system does not need nourishment at the time. Let the patient drink freely of pure, soft cold water ; this will be found to support the strength wonderfully, and with such a course, other circumstances also being favorable, the stomach will retain food as soon as the system needs nourishing.

Vomiting in pregnancy has been known not unfrequently to be so exceedingly severe, as to cause abortion. So also practitioners have regarded it their duty to bring on premature labor or abortion, hoping thereby to save the life of the mother, which they regarded as being in imminent danger from the vomiting I should be glad to see the case of this kind that could withstand prolonged fasting, water-drinking, and bathing, if such a case could be found. In vomiting, both patients and physicians seem to be afraid of nothing so much as starvation. Hence the stomach is made the receptacle of all manner of things, clean and unclean, saying nothing of the inordinate dosing that is usually practiced on such occasions. It is no wonder that the vomiting continues under such treatment.

With correct general habits, let the patient who is so much troubled with vomiting, confine herself to one article of food, as good brown bread and water, and the difficulty dies away. Dr. Dewees tells us that he had known the best effects occur from substituting a glass of cold water for tea or coffee in the morning, by which the patients were enabled to retain a cracker or two on the stomach, which would not have been the case, had they taken either of the other substances. He also mentions the case of one lady, who could keep nothing at all on the stomach, except Indian meal cakes, baked on a board, which she literally lived upon for weeks. Causing a free movement of the bowels by one or two full injections of cold water, will be found to have a very excellent effect in arresting vomiting.

When bilious and acid matters are vomited, the drinking of a large quantity of blood-warm water quickly, so as to cause a thorough cleansing of the stomach, should be practiced.

It should be mentioned here, that people often err in these cases of excessive vomiting, by taking too much food at a time. A tea-spoonfull of milk or gruel, or a piece of bread the size of a walnut, well chewed and swallowed, could hardly be vomited up at all. By beginning nourishment thus gradually, persons may often subdue the most obstinate vomiting.

MORBID CRAVING FOR FOOD.

Women sometimes experience in pregnancy, cravings for strange and unnatural things to eat, such not unfrequently as they would utterly loathe at other times. Those who suffer from indigestion, those who have constipation, and especially those who are hysterical, experience these morbid cravings.

In some parts of the country, and in cities too, we

suppose, it is thought by many dangerous not to gratify these longings. Not only has it been supposed that the unborn infant might be injured, if the mother's fancies are not gratified, but even that the mark of the thing longed for is likely to be impressed upon it.

This, like many other things, goes no doubt very much by fashion. Many ignorant, nervous women, seem to suppose that it is really a necessary part of their being to have these longings in pregnancy.

We need hardly say that these longings should never be gratified. No possible good can come from it; only harm, the same as at other times.

PAIN IN THE RIGHT SIDE.

After gestation has passed the middle of its term, there is experienced often more or less pain in the right side. This does not usually happen until after the beginning of the fifth month of pregnancy. It comes on as a deep-seated pain in the immediate region of the liver; often it is merely a trifling sensation at first, increasing as pregnancy advances. It is not increased by ordinary inspirations, as many internal pains are, although a very full and deep inspiration may augment it in a slight degree. The pain is seldom, almost never, very great; it is constant both day and night, but worse in the latter. The patient can lie on either side, but better on the left. A severe sensation of heat is sometimes experienced at the part where the pain exists. This is sometimes almost constant, at others only occasional, and in still a greater number of instances nothing of the kind occurs. Women are more subject to this affection during the first pregnancy than at subsequent times. It may, how-

7

ever, be experienced after a number of children have
been borne; this is true more especially in those cases
when the child is carried "high up," as it is called.
This comes from the fact, that the pain is caused by the
pressure of the upper part of the womb upon the liver,
which lies mostly upon the right side.

No material harm can be said to come from this pain,
and for this reason no harsh and severe medical treatment should be adopted with a view of removing it.
Bleeding is well known to be a common remedy for ordinary pains in the side. But Dr. Dewees, of Philadelphia, whose experience was so great in all matters pertaining to midwifery, remarks of this practice, that so
far as he had seen it, not the slightest advantage had
arisen from it. "Nor," observes this candid writer,
"has any other treatment which we have advised been
any more successful. Leeching, cupping, and blistering,
have in turn been employed without benefit. Indeed, we
have now ceased to prescribe for this complaint, unless
it be attended with some alteration in the circulating system if this be disturbed, and the pulse tense and frequent, advantage is sometimes experienced from the loss
of blood and gentle purging, as this pain may be aggravated by this condition of the system. But in this instance, we prescribe for the general condition of the
system, and not for the local affection—as we should
have to do most probably as much, were this pain in
the side not present." These are the candid remarks
of one whose experience in treating diseases of women
was as great, probably, as that of any other man,
showing conclusively that ordinary means are of no
avail in this difficulty

Now I can speak confidently in this matter   The

water processes are effectual in mitigating this pain much, to say the least. I conclude it is rather a symptom of debility than otherwise. I do not believe it natural. Bathing to support the general strength, and particularly the wet girdle often rewet, especially in hot weather, so as to keep it at all times cool, and hip baths, with a good share of friction by the wet hand over the part affected, will be found excellent means. The *immediate* relief caused by the application of the wet girdle will be often astonishing. Keeping the bowels freely open, as by the habitual use of brown bread, mush, and the like, and injections of cold water, are also of service here.

But if, in any case, the pain resists all remedial means, and as we have before said, those of a severe nature should never be resorted to, the individual should not allow her mind to become depressed by thinking that harm must inevitably be caused in consequence of it Such is by no means the case.

Too much as well as too little exercise may cause this difficulty. A proper medium should therefore at all times be observed.

CONSTIPATION.

During the early months of pregnancy, there appears to be a greater tendency to constipation than in the latter months, a fact which is the direct reverse of what we should expect from *a priori* reasoning. But during the whole period, constipation is more apt to occur than at other times.

Constipation is exceedingly common among all classes of females in this country at the present day. The

American people have such a predilection for fine food it is a hard matter to make any great change in this respect. It is in the dietetic habits more than in any other that we are to look for the causes of this evil.

Superfine flour is, I hold, the greatest of all causes of constipation. I know tea and coffee, which are astringent articles, have a tendency to cause this condition of the bowels ; and the same may be said of idleness and physical inactivity ; but too great richness in food— and superfine flour is the article most consumed in this— is the great cause of constipation. Our country abounds with it every where. By our numerous railroads and canals, superfine flour is transported from one end of the country to the other, so that in large districts where formerly the people were in the habit of eating coarse bread, as of rye and Indian, and were consequently more healthy, they now use the superfine. Even a beggar would sneer at one for offering him brown bread.

Constipation, common as it is every where among females, is still more common in pregnancy. This arises, first, from the pressure of the enlarged womb upon the lower bowel ; and second, there being a new action set up in the uterus, there is, as a natural consequence, a greater tendency to torpor in the bowels. But the principal cause is that of the pressure.

This condition of the bowels induces of itself numerous other difficulties. Headache is often brought on solely by constipation ; that is, in many cases we remove the constipation, and the headache is sure to leave with it. Sickness of the stomach and vomiting are always aggravated, and often caused by it. The same also may be said of heart-burn, palpitation, and fainting. Sleeplessness, and in fact almost every one of the disorders of pregnancy, may be said to be either caused directly or greatly aggravated by constipation of the bowels. Even miscarriage has been known to be induced by it.

Some persons have gone almost an incredible length of time without any movement of the bowels. A whole week is not uncommon. Dr. Dewees mentions a case of fourteen days, and no doubt there have been those who have gone one to three whole weeks.

What have we to do in order to cure constipation of the bowels? Does not every person of common sense understand at this day, that the more we dose the sys tem for constipation the more we may? Let those answer who have tried these things. Always, other things being equal, the more we take drugs for constipation the worse it grows. We must therefore look to some other means of cure.

Constipation of the bowels may always be cured, and this by the most simple means. Dr. Dewees mentions a case where a lady had suffered three successive miscarriages from this cause, and by the constant use of brown bread, drinking only water, and taking no animal food or broths—taking now and then a little castor oil or the like, which, however, he did not reckon upon as having done any material good—enabled her to pass safely through the whole time. We need here only mention, in general terms, that constipation in pregnancy is to be cured just the same as constipation in any other case. Brown bread, fruits, and vegetables, with a very moderate use of milk, if the patient desires it; regular exercise, the hip bath, wet girdle, injections of cold water, or tepid, if that is preferred—these are the means to be used. The brown wheat or rye mush

7*

will be found most excellent. No woman, if she can Have brown bread, and occasionally an injection, need ever suffer from constipation of the bowels.

DIARRHŒA.

Sometimes the reverse of constipation occurs during pregnancy; namely, diarrhœa. This also not unfrequently alternates with constipation. Constipation, however, is the most frequent symptom.

Singular as it may appear, diarrhœa should be treated on the same general principles as constipation. Fortify and invigorate the general health, observing at the same time a correct general regimen, and either symptom disappears. In diarrhœa, the hip bath, often repeated, the wet girdle, and cold injections, taken as often as there is any disposition for the bowels to act, are effectual means. The diet should be regulated on the strictest principles. If a diarrhœa is very severe, entire abstinence from all nourishment except water for a day or two, is a very salutary remedy. Food should then be taken with the same precautions as in nausea and vomiting.

PILES AND HÆMORRHOIDS.

Piles and hæmorrhoids are more apt to occur in pregnancy than at other times; and when these already existed, they are apt to become worse at this period. Constipation being more apt to occur in pregnancy, and that condition of the system being the one in which these symptoms are most liable to occur when the woman is not pregnant, so also they occur more frequently now than at other times. The constant pressure of the fœtus upon the blood-vessels within the pelvis has also an agency in the matter, because every thing that causes sluggishness of circulation tends to bring on piles. So also the more sedentary habits of many females during the period of pregnancy, are often a cause of this difficulty ; but in other cases the opposite extreme is practiced—too much exercise or standing on the feet. Both these extremes may cause piles in pregnancy, or aggravation when they previously existed. Cathartic medicines not unfrequently bring on a "fit of the piles."

This affection always denotes a wrong state of things in the general health. A really healthy person can never have the piles. Some, however, who are what would be termed tolerably well and strong in general health, experience such symptoms ; but such is not the rule. Old cases, particularly, denote derangement of the general system.

When piles come suddenly, they are often attended with very great pain and suffering to the patient. Not only is the pain great at the part affected, but there is also feverishness, pain, and a very unpleasant feeling in the head, with deep and severe pain in the back.

As to the treatment and general management in this affection, we should of course do the best that may be for the general health. As a general fact, no surgical operation should be allowed upon piles during pregnancy. These operations are often attended with so great pain, that abortion might be the result.

There is nothing in the world that will produce so great relief in piles as fasting. If the fit is severe, live a whole day (or even two, if necessary) upon pure, soft cold water alone. Give then very lightly of vegetable food. Those who have suffered the agony of this affection, if they will but have patience to try this means will find the truth of my remarks.

Water applications are also very useful in this disease. Dr. Dewees observes : " The pregnant woman may derive both comfort and advantage from sitting in a demibath of cold water for five or ten minutes at a time two or three times a day, when the complaint is advancing, or when about to retire ; that is, after the severer symptoms have abated, or before they are high." This advice is partly right and partly not. There is a notion with many that cold water applications in high inflammation are not good ; that they increase the difficulty instead of making it less. Thus in a burn, it is said that after the application of cold water the pain becomes worse. This is not true, although it appears to be so ; for so great is the relief afforded by the application, that the pain *appears* to be worse, when in fact it is not. But only keep on continuously with the cold water treatment, and the pain does not return at all. Such at least is the fact in all burns, however severe, when the surface is not destroyed ; and the same principle holds good in all high inflammations from whatever cause. Very frequent sitz baths, or merely washing the piles often in cold water, will be found excellent in those severe cases of piles. Cold compresses worn upon the part, also afford great relief. Cold injections are also useful. But, as before mentioned, *fasting and the regulation of the diet* are the great means.

ITCHING OF THE GENITAL ORGANS.

Pruritus pudendi, or itching of the genital parts, becomes sometimes a most troublesome and distressing complaint in pregnancy ; so troublesome, indeed, as utterly to set decency at defiance. Cases under the ordinary modes of treatment, have been known to be so severe as to compel the lady to remain in her chamber for months.

The causes of this affection cannot always be ascertained. A want of proper cleanliness is no doubt often one of the principal sources of it.

A great variety of remedial means have been used in this disease. Astringents, such as alum, borax, acids, etc., are the agents indicated. But cold is the greatest astringent of all ; no matter how troublesome the affection, it is completely within our control by the use of cold hip baths, cold cloths, ice, and the like. In a late number of *Braithwait's Retrospect*, one of the leading English periodicals of medicine and surgery, it is stated by Dr. James Arnott, " that a most distressing attack of this affection was completely subdued by two congelations, each of about thirty seconds' duration, after a prussic acid lotion and other routine applications had been tried in vain." By " congelation," Dr. Arnott means the application of intense cold, by the use of ice between cloths, or some freezing mixture, but not an actual freezing of the parts, as some might suppose. But shallow hip baths of cold water from a well, persevered in, will be found sufficient in every case.

SWELLINGS OF THE LIMBS AND VARICOSE VEINS.

Swellings of the lower limbs, and varicose or knotty and swelled veins, may occur in pregnancy from the same causes as piles and hæmorrhoids, namely, au obstructed circulation.

Washing the parts affected with cold water, and attention to the general health, are the means to be used here. Do no violence to the system. The exercise should be moderate. Nor should the woman be too inactive; the medium course in all cases is the better rule.

CRAMPS IN THE LOWER LIMBS.

Toward the close of pregnancy, cramps may occur in the lower extremities, because of the pressure of the child upon the large nerves that pass down them. This is seldom very troublesome, and cannot of course be altogether prevented. Too great fatigue, and any thing that tends to depress the general health, will at least make the matter worse than it otherwise would be.

PAIN IN THE BREASTS.

Mastodynia, or pain in the breasts, is more common in the first pregnancy. Compression by clothing may cause the difficulty. Washing the parts with cold water, and wet bandages or cloths worn upon the parts, are the means to be used. If the pain is of a spasmodic kind, it may be best in some cases to use warm fomentations.

URINARY DIFFICULTIES.

Incontinence of urine is quite apt to occur toward the end of pregnancy. It arises often from the pressure of the child upon the neck of the bladder. There is a notion with some of the "old women," that incontinence of urine is an indication of good labor. This difficulty cannot of course be altogether remedied; the cause cannot be removed. It may be lessened, however, by short and frequent hip baths, wet bandages, and cold bathing. Drinking soft water instead of hard, will also be found to have a good effect in all difficulties of the bladder whatever.

Blisters are always liable to bring trouble upon the urinary organs, but more particularly so in pregnancy. The system is then in a more excitable or impressible state. Strangury in pregnancy is a very distressing and untoward symptom when it follows the use of blisters. Dr. Dewees had known cases where entire retention of urine followed the use of blisters, so obstinate that it could only be relieved by the catheter, causing a distressing inclination and violence of effort only o be surpassed by labor itself.

Retention may also come on from other causes. As to the treatment, it can be very seldom indeed necessary to resort to the use of the catheter for draining off the urine, if cold hip baths, cold foot baths, and even the cold general bath, if necessary, be sufficiently persevered in. Cold has a truly wonderful effect in causing the flow of urine.

THE MIND AS AFFECTED BY PREGNANCY.

The mind not unfrequently becomes materially affected during pregnancy. But there is a remarkable difference among women in this particular ; some become cross, fretful, peevish, and irritable, and even passionate, while with others the mental health seems in no way disturbed, and in some instances becomes actually improved. Considering what the physical education of females has been, and with the many still is—faulty and erroneous in almost every thing—we should not find fault with them if the mind does become unpleasantly affected during the state of pregnancy. I would not in the least excuse the exceeding passionateness which some allow themselves to exhibit during this period, evidently without cause; but I would only inculcate a proper degree of leniency and consideration in those cases where such are evidently demanded. Be it remarked, also, that when the individual has been reared according to the true principles of physiological science, and continues to practice regularly and consistently in accordance therewith, little need be feared from mental disturbance during the period of pregnancy.

HYSTERIA IN PREGNANCY.

There appears to be with many a greater tendency to hysterical symptoms during pregnancy than at other times. Hysterical females are for the most part those who live a life of excitement, attending frequently balls, theatres, and public exhibitions late at night, and especially such as are much addicted to tea and coffee drinking, the use of concentrated and stimulating food, and have little exercise in the open air. Medicines, especially the preparations of opium, also have a tendency to cause hysterical symptoms. Pregnant women should, then, as far as possible, avoid these causes of so pitiable a disease. Whether in pregnancy or at other times, hysteria cannot come upon those who live correctly, and maintain at all times good and permanent health. I will here further remark, that all novel-reading should be avoided during pregnancy; and the less the better, I may say, at all times, of such novels as ninety-nine hundredths of all that are put forth at the present day.

CHAPTER VI.

MISCARRIAGE OR ABORTION, AND BARRENNESS.

Miscarriage or Abortion becoming more common at the present day.—The reasons why.—Rules to be Observed.—What Females are most liable to Abortion.—Vile Books concerning Abortion.—Means of Preventing it.—Cold Water an excellent Remedy.—Feather Beds and Pillows injurious.—Vegetable Diet better than Animal.—Hæmorrhage from the womb in Pregnancy not necessarily attended with Abortion.—Abortion generally a more serious matter than Labor at full term.—Those who miscarry once are more apt to do so again.—Very feeble Persons should not become Pregnant.—The treatment in Miscarriage.—What to do in the absence of a Physician.—Cold a better means than Blood-letting for arresting Uterine Hæmorrhage.—Barrenness.—Bathing and Diet often effectual in this matter.

MISCARRIAGE OR ABORTION.

MISCARRIAGES are becoming more and more common in this country. A principal reason for this is, that the habits of a great part of the community are less in accordance with physiological principles than was formerly the case. It is not *fashionable* now-a-days to spin and weave, and do many kinds of useful work, as it was in the days of our grandmothers. Besides, people are growing more indolent. The sluggard will not plow by reason of the cold ; he shall therefore beg in harvest and have nothing. So also those who will not use the limbs and muscles which God has given them, cannot have health at any price.

I would have my daughters taught music, painting, drawing, as well as the useful sciences, but on no account at the expense of bodily health. Nor is there

8

need of this; for the highest possible cultivation of the mental powers can only be accomplished when the physical powers are suitably and proportionably developed. "A sound mind in a sound body" is the law.

Females cannot be too careful of their bodily health during pregnancy, if they would avoid the misfortune of abortion. A little imprudence here, such as would scarcely be noticed at other times, may lay the foundation for much future suffering. I am here led to remark, that too much labor and exercise, as well as idleness and habits of effeminacy, not unfrequently cause miscarriage. Idle people do too little; industrious people often too much.

Fat women, and those who experience excessive menstruation; those who are hysterical, nervous, irritable, or excessively sensitive; those who have a very fair complexion, and are rickety, scrofulous, or have any other taint of the general system; those who have dropsy, or are affected with cancer; and especially those who compress their bodies with stays, corsets, or other tight clothing; and above all, those who, by reason of their sensual, and worse than brutish husbands, abuse the marital privileges, are most apt to suffer miscarriages. If husbands have any regard for the health of either their wives or their offspring, let them refrain from all sexual indulgences during the period of pregnancy.*

* DR. EDWARD BAYNARD, an able and very sarcastic English writer, one hundred and fifty years ago, in speaking of the evil effects of swathing and dressing infants too tightly, indulged in the following reflections: "'Tis a great shame that greater care is not taken in so weighty an affair, as is the birth and breeding of that noble creature, MAN; and, considering this stupid and supine negligence, I have often wondered that there are so many men as there are in the world: for what by abortions too oft

Terror, fright, and excessive fatigue, as before said, may cause abortion. All unpleasant sights, and all undue mental excitements, should be most scrupulously avoided by those who are pregnant.

There are vile books in circulation, sold too, sometimes, by highly respectable booksellers, in which the writers affirm that abortion can be produced *without any harm to the constitution.* There is one physician in this city, whose book we saw a few days since in a bookstore in the city of Boston, in which he proposes to effect abortion with perfect safety but for the package of medicine a fee of *ten dollars* must be sent, of course, in advance. It may be of service to some who may peruse these pages, for me to inform them that there is always great danger in causing the expulsion of the fœtus. The most powerful medicines for this purpose are often known to fail. Gastritis, enteritis, peritonitis, and death itself has been caused by medication, without causing the intended abortion.

PREVENTION OF ABORTION.

Cold bathing, for its tonic and constringing effect, has for centuries been recommended as a most valuable means of preventing abortion. In pregnancy, the same general principles should be observed in fortifying and invigorating the general health as at other times. No violence should be done to the system. A general bath

caused by the unseasonable, too frequent, and boisterous, drunken addresses of the husband to the wife, when young with child, and her high feeding, spiced meats, soups, and sauces, which with strait lacings, dancings, and the like, one full half of the men begotten are destroyed in the shell, squabed in the nest, murdered in embryo, and never see light; and half of the other half are overlaid, poisoned by ill food, and killed at nurse," etc.

in the morning, cool or cold, according to the individual's strength; a hip or sitz bath of five or ten minutes' duration. two or three times during the day, and an ablution with water, not too cold, on going to rest, will ordinarily be sufficient for the daily routine of treatment in those cases where there is tendency to abortion; such a course is in fact good at all times. The wet girdle, elsewhere explained, will often be of advantage; but to make it a tonic or strengthening application, as it should always be under these circumstances, great care must be taken that it does not become too warm. This is very apt to be the case in hot weather. It must then be changed often and rewet. If it becomes too hot, it weakens the system instead of strengthening it, thus tending to cause the very difficulty it is intended to prevent. "Injecting cold water into the vagina, twice or thrice a day," says Dr. Burns, in his work on midwifery, "has often a good effect, at the same time that we continue the shower bath." And this writer also observes, "that when there is much aching pain in the back, it is of service to apply cloths to it, dipped in cold water, or gently to dash cold water on it, or employ a partial shower bath, by means of a small watering can." Water, let it be remembered, is the greatest of all tonics to the living system.

Sleeping upon feather beds and in overheated rooms has much to do in causing abortions. People ought never to sleep on a feather bed, unless, possibly, very old and feeble persons who have long been accustomed to them. In such cases it might not always be safe to make a change in cold weather suddenly. But for a pregnant women to sleep on a feather bed is one of the worst of practices. And here also I must mention that feather pillows, as well as feather beds, do a great amount of harm. Even those who have emancipated themselves from the evils of feather beds, usually retain the feather pillow. It is a wise old maxim, "to keep the head cool." The head has blood enough, more than any other part of the system, to keep it warm. No person, not even the youngest infant, should ever sleep on a bed or pillow made of feathers. The animal effluvia coming from them is bad, and the too great amount of heat retained about the surface debilitates the system in every respect.

The vegetable diet was observed by the celebrated Dr. Cheyne, of England, to have a great influence in preventing abortions. Milk, however, was generally used, which is in some sense animal food. A total milk and seed diet, as Dr. Cheyne terms it, was a most excellent means of preventing infertility and abortion.

Hæmorrhage from the womb, during the months of pregnancy, is not necessarily attended with abortion. Great care, however, should be exercised if hæmorrhage occur during this period, as there is then always great danger of losing the child.

Abortion, as a general fact, is a more serious matter than birth at the full period. Hippocrates asserted that a miscarriage is generally more dangerous than a labor at full term. The reason of this is, the first is an unnatural occurrence; the second natural. In many instances, however, the abortion itself is of far less consequence than the condition of the general health which allows of such an occurrence. For the most part it is only the feeble and debilitated that experience abortions.

Women who miscarry once, are much more apt to do so again. The body, like the mind, appears to have a

8*

great tendency to get into bad habits; and the older the habit the worse it becomes, and the more difficult of control.

It were better for very feeble persons not to place themselves in the way of becoming pregnant; certainly not until the general health has been attended to. And it is a fortunate thing for society that many feeble and diseased persons are wholly incapable of begetting off-spring; otherwise the race would soon run out.

More than one hundred years ago, the celebrated Dr. Cheyne remarked concerning abortion and its causes as follows: "It is a vulgar error to confine tender-breeding women to their chambers, couches, or beds during all the time of their pregnancy. This is one of the readiest ways to make them miscarry. It is like the common advice of some unskillful persons to such as have anasarcous or dropsical legs, namely, to keep them up in chairs on a level with their seats, which is the ready way to throw up the humors into their bowels and fix them there. The only solid and certain way to prevent miscarriage, is to pursue all those means and methods that are the likeliest to procure or promote good health, of which air and gentle exercise are one of the principal. All violence or excesses of every kind are to be carefully avoided by the parturient; but fresh air, gentle exercise, walking, being carried in a sedan or chaise on even ground, is as necessary as food or rest; and therefore is never to be omitted, when the season will permit, by tender breeders."

TREATMENT IN ABORTION.

The limits of this work will not admit of my entering into a long explanation of the different modes of treatment in the various stages of abortion. Nor is it the design of the author to undertake to teach people how to get along without the aid of a physician, male or female, who has given these important subjects proper consideration. There are certain things, however, which people generally can and ought of themselves to do. It often happens, moreover, that no medical adviser can be obtained immediately ; and for this reason, also, people ought to inform themselves of the best modes of arresting hæmorrhage, the thing mainly to be attended to in abortion.

When abortion is about to take place, the woman experiences usually for some time previously, " a sense of weight and weakness in the loins and region of the uterus, followed by stitches of pain shooting through the lower part of the abdomen, back, and thighs." There may be also bearing-down pains in the bowels, and frequent desire to pass urine. In connection with these symptoms—that is, at or about the same time—the discharge of blood commences. This is sometimes so sudden and rapid, that the strength becomes very soon exhausted to a great degree. If much blood passes, abortion is almost certain to take place.

Bleeding, for its sedative, is often resorted to on these occasions. The application of cold, however, is the more effectual means when suitably made. Cold, as well as bleeding, is a sedative ; and besides being as powerful as we choose to make it, has this great advantage over bleeding—it does not reduce the strength

It performs the effect without robbing the patient of that important agent, the blood.

In any case of hæmorrhage from the womb, then, persons should, in the absence of a physician, at once resort to the application of cold.   There is heat and feverishness in the system, be it remembered; under such circumstances it is impossible to "take cold," of which people are every where so much afraid.   Cold wet cloths, often changed, should be applied about the abdomen, upon the genital parts, thighs, etc.   Use plenty of cloths, and even doubled sheets, dipped in the coldest water. A piece of ice, wrapped within a cloth, is also often put up the vagina for a little time, to produce a chilling effect.   Until the bleeding stops, it is next thing to impossible to do any harm with cold.   Cold injections to the bowels and vagina, and when the patient is not too weak, the cold hip bath, are useful means.   "A rigid avoidance of every thing stimulating; a cool room; cool drinks; and light bed-clothes," are recommended by Dr. Maunsel.

After the bleeding has ceased, the patient should be allowed to rest, and she should be nursed in the most careful manner.   For days and weeks, and, in some cases, for whole months, the greatest care must be exercised, lest a little overdoing, a little excitement, or some other untoward circumstance, may bring injury upon the patient.

BARRENNESS.

Barrenness should be mentioned in connection with abortion.   Some two years ago, I wrote in my notebook as follows:

"A few months since, one of my patients, a gentleman

of this city, informed me that a lady relative of his, with whom also I am acquainted, had been married about eight years, remaining, much to her sorrow, childless. She experienced frequent miscarriages, accompanied with much general debility. About two years since, the subject of water-treatment came under her observation. She at once commenced a course of bathing, with due attention to regimen, etc. She became much improved, and, in due time, bore a healthy, well-formed child. She attributed this most desirable result to the effects of water in restoring her general health.

" Another lady remained without offspring for fifteen years after marriage Her husband, in building a new house since the introduction of Croton water into this city, erected also convenient bathing fixtures. The lady practiced perseveringly a course of bathing, and became much improved in her bodily health. She too was at length blessed with an offspring, and, as she believed, in consequence of the course she had pursued in restoring her general health.

"I have known and heard of numbers of cases in which, by a prudent course of bathing, exercise, etc., the use of a plain and unstimulating diet, and the observing of proper temperance in the marital privileges, persons have borne children when most earnestly, and by a great variety of means, that object had been sought in vain. Yet be it ever remembered, that little is to be expected from either water or diet without *strict temperance in all things.*"

The vegetable diet, so called, is very favorable to reproduction in the human species. See how Ireland, a small island comparatively, sends its inhabitants all over Great Britain and the wide extent of the United States

Yet the mass of Irish people, as every one knows, subsist, while in their own country, mainly on potatoes and sour milk, or a diet equally simple. The celebrated Dr. Cheyne remarked, from much experience, that the total milk and seed diet (meaning by seed, farinaceous substances generally), persevered in for two years, was in almost all cases sufficient to enable the barren to become pregnant by the appropriate means.

Fortify and invigorate the general health, observing at the same time the strictest "temperance in all things." These are the means by which to overcome that, to many, unfortunate state, **barrenness.**

CHAPTER VII.

CASES OF CHILDBIRTH.

" *July 5th,* 1848.—Mrs. Webster, age 38, was born ot healthy parents in the state of Rhode Island, and when young had a good constitution. Somewhere early in her teens she became feeble. Every body laced in those times, *i. e.,* the ladies, and it were a wonder if she did not. About her eighteenth year, she was treated for what was termed spinal disease, and so onward for three years. She was at one time confined to her bed for fifteen months. During this time she had drawn from her, by cupping, leeching, and bleeding, some gallons of blood. No wonder she was weak, nervous, discouraged. By cuppings, scarifications, burnings, cauterizations, moxas, etc., the whole region from the neck to below the small of the back, was made almost one perfect mass of scar.

" At length, with the spinal disease yet upon her, she was attacked with the typhus fever, receiving it apparently from a brother who died of it. She had a long time of it, and barely escaped death. With this sickness the spinal disease left her. All along during that disease Mrs. Webster's good mother, of wealthy family, and a real Howard among the sick, prepared for her the finest of beef-steaks, swimming in butter, oysters, fine bread, buttered toast, and all manner of the richest things conceivable.

"Good mothers do not let their daughters suffer for any thing in the world they think will do them good. No wonder she had typhus fever after all the drugging, bleeding, and abominable diet. The wonder is that she lived at all.

"After a few years all the old symptoms of the spinal complaint returned upon her. She now fell into Dr. Webster's hands for the first time, when he gave her some weeks of Thomsonian treatment. This apparently worked wonders for her.

"Since marriage, three years ago, Mrs. Webster has experienced a number of miscarriages, early ones all of them; the first was caused by being thrown from a horse. Two years ago this July (1848), she gave birth to her first child. Under the good care of her husband she got up very well; but her infant died when ten weeks old. This affliction proved a terrible one for her, and her health became very much depressed by it. After this there were one or more miscarriages.

"About the first of October, 1847, she became again pregnant. Twenty-three days since, just as Mrs. Webster and husband were coming to remain awhile with us at Oyster Bay, she was attacked with what at first appeared like canker in the mouth. It resulted, however, in an erysipelatous inflammation of the mouth and one side of the face. The swelling broke in the mouth about ten days after the attack.

"Eleven days since Dr. W. and wife arrived at our establishment, she expecting to be confined in two or three weeks. She could walk but little; going a short distance fatigued her much. Doctor Webster applied the water faithfully and exclusively during the attack of the erysipelas mentioned, so that she was gaining fast when she came. A worthy and so called intelligent cousin of hers in Providence, said to Dr. Webster, the night of leaving, ' *You are killing your wife,*' and· thought, no doubt, she would never return alive.

" TREATMENT AT OYSTER BAY.—Rubbing sheet, of rain-water temperature, say about 70 degrees Fah., on rising in the morning, usually at about four o'clock. Then she walked in the open air, wet or dry, when it did not actually rain in torrents. She drank also some water always after the bath, during the walks and after returning to her room. This exercise in the open air, practiced moderately at first, together with the baths, proved a great tonic to the system. She walked at different times of the day, when the sun was not too hot, mostly mornings and evenings. In the hot part of the forenoon she rested on the bed, and generally obtained some good sleep. This, however, she could not have done had not the clothing been removed as at going to rest at night. Persons wonder how it is that when they sleep in the day time they wake up so feverish and unrefreshed. Keeping the clothing on never does well in sleep.

" *Forenoon.*—After resting, and from half an hour to an hour before dinner, the rubbing sheet was applied as in the morning. Feet were washed at the same time. She in fact always stood in a tub having water in it two or three inches deep, of rain-water temperature. She was to wash the feet at any time when they felt hot and disagreeable ; so also the hands and face.

" *Afternoon.*—The rubbing sheet toward supper time as before dinner. Was to keep up in the afternoon and avoid sleeping, so that the rest at night would not be disturbed.

9

"*Evening.*—At about nine o'clock, and on going to rest, the rubbing sheet and foot-washing as before. Hip baths, one or two inches deep, were to be taken at any time when there were itchings, heat, etc., causing a need for them.

"*Food.*—Vegetable food and fruits, with a moderate portion of good milk, constituted her diet. No other drink than water was used. The meals were taken between six and seven A. M., twelve M., and six P. M. There was no eating between times as people are wont to do ; appetite and enjoyment of food were remarkably good ; no meals omitted.

"Remarks on the Rubbing Sheet.—This was applied with good, strong, old-fashioned linen. Quite dripping wet, it was put upon the shoulders and about the whole body in the standing posture ; moderate friction was made (*over* the sheet, not *with* it) for about five minutes. The body was then made dry with towels. A few times, when Mrs. W. felt very languid, Dr. Webster applied the sheet twice in succession. This always revived her very sensibly. When she had the erysipelas before coming to us, Dr. Webster usually poured water upon the wet sheet while it was yet upon the body, and after the rubbing had made it somewhat warm ; and after this, rubbing was practiced again to excite a glow.

"Under the above treatment Mrs. W. gained strength remarkably ; soon became able to walk two and a half miles in the morning. She slept in a large and well-ventilated room, and her rest was uniformly good.

"*Confinement.*—The third of July was one of her best days. She slept remarkably well at night, even better than common, as if nature, in anticipation of the coming event, were recruiting her energies to the utmost.

Rose at half past four; then the pains commenced very slightly; took the rubbing sheet and an injection, and thought she would walk out; but the pains grew steadily worse till half past eight o'clock, when her infant, a large and healthy male child, was born. The labor was very easy; almost nothing compared with the former one. In about three quarters of an hour the after-birth was expelled. Wet towels were kept upon the genital organs and the abdomen, and changed often enough to prevent their becoming too warm. So also common sense would dictate that a patient should not be too much chilled at such a time, and yet there is here a great amount of unnecessary fear respecting cold applications. There is incomparably more to be feared from the effects of feather beds, close rooms, bad food and drinks, bandages, etc., in general use.

"After the birth, Mrs. Webster slept well awhile, and at noon she had a thorough ablution as follows: In a hip bath-tub (a common wash-tub of middling size is good), a bucket of cold, soft well water was put, and then moderated with hot water to about 70 degrees Fah. Dr. Webster aided her in rising, and she bore her own weight both before and after the bath. She sat in the tub for some fifteen minutes, a blanket being about the body; the whole body was thoroughly washed during this time; the water, she said, was exceedingly refreshing. Afterward the hands and face were washed in the cold water.

"After resting half an hour she ate dinner with an excellent appetite, for she had had no breakfast. The meal was a very plain one, viz., a small piece of brown bread toast, with a few good uncooked whortleberries. Gin s.ing, toddy, tea, coffee, and other s ops which are brought into requisition on such occasions, have no place, it will be remembered, in our Water Vocabulary. After the bath, as well as after the dinner, our patient felt remarkably well, quite as much so as any one ; now and then there were slight after-pains. She sat up at different times in the afternoon, being up and lying down alternately as she felt inclined, possessing too much knowledge and good sense to be carried away with the foolish nine day whims of society.

"At between six and seven of this day it would have been well for Mrs. W. to have had another bath, but Dr. Webster being absent, it was omitted ; then also a third bath between nine and ten on going to rest. Meal at evening same as at noon, with the exception of the bread being moistened with milk. After sundown she sat up two hours at least. The evening bath was as refreshing as at noon, and aided much in procuring good rest. The ignorant people may yet learn something of the good and the safety of these applications scientifically made.

"*Second day.*—Patient slept remarkably well until about two o'clock. Then there came on after-pains, and the infant made some noise, which circumstances together kept her awake part of the time. Here the bath should have been given, which would have prevented the pains, and caused good sleep. Very early in the morning she arose and took the ablution as the day before. She felt well and strong ; walked about her room. We should have mentioned she walked also the previous evening. Breakfast same as the supper. After this she walked down stairs with a little aid from her husband, entered a carriage and rode with him a full hour and a half. This pleasant ride in the cool of the morning was to her exceedingly refreshing; she was not fatigued, only made better for it. Knowing it would be so was the reason of our directing it.

"Awhile after returning from the ride, she laid down and slept soundly. Before dinner she took again her accustomed bath. Dinner, green peas without butter or salt, with brown bread, and a few good raspberries uncooked.

"At evening, between six and seven, Mrs. W. again rode out. Was up more than two thirds of the entire day; experienced some pains; these were each time mitigated by the bath. The ablutions are performed regularly on rising, before dinner, before supper, on going to rest, and in the night time if the after-pains become troublesome. A good deal of friction with the hand at the time of, and after the bath. Injections of cold water, to which she has been accustomed, are used daily. The morning, before breakfast, is perhaps the best time. They may be taken a number of times during the day if the pains are severe. One or two pints may be used. If the patient is very weak they should not be too cold, 70 degrees F. being a good temperature.

"*Third day.*—Mrs. W. slept not very well. Invalids seldom, if ever, sleep right well more than one or two nights in succession. She feels, however, remarkably well, and is gaining strength rapidly every day: bathes, sits up, walks, and rides as usual. She could now return home to Providence without risk, were it necessary for her to do so.

"When cases like the above in water-treatment are spoken of by friends of the system, objectors, especially the doctors, at once say, 'Did you never hear of poor

Irish women getting up immediately and going to the wash-tub?' Let it be understood, now and ever, *we ask only that the rule of our cases be taken as the test.* We give such examples as are an *average* of our success under this treatment."

The above case was thus written out for the Water-Cure Journal soon after it occurred. Within two or three months after the birth of the child, Mrs. Webster was again attacked slightly with erysipelas, but this was readily managed as before. It is now about eight months since her infant was born, and both she and it have enjoyed, with little exception, remarkably good health. It was said by some objectors to the water-treatment at Oyster Bay, not over-modestly, " that Mrs. Webster must be some strong Irish or Scotch woman whom Dr. Shew had got to show off with." The case, as given above, will speak for itself; and it is proper for me here to remark, that Mrs. Webster is at least not behind *any* of the ladies of Oyster Bay in intelligence, good manners, and education ; and the only reason—I repeat, the *only* reason—why she allows her name to be used in this public manner is, that she has none of that *false modesty* which causes persons to shrink from any thing, the promulgation of which may be of good to the human race.

CASE II.

A few weeks after the case of Mrs. Webster, I attended the wife of a clergyman at Oyster Bay, whose name I presume there would be no objection to my using ; but as I have not obtained the liberty, it would not be proper to do it. The lady, Mrs. R., is of about the same age of Mrs. Webster, of very good constitution, but ha

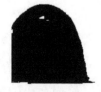

bits too sedentary. Some years before she had borne one child, which was her first. She had at that time a long four weeks' siege of getting up, that very naturally made her dread the second accouchement. Eight or nine weeks, perhaps more, before the birth, she commenced bathing pretty systematically. She attended daily to her household affairs, but seldom walked out.

Labor came on one Saturday afternoon, lasting only about two hours, when it terminated favorably in the birth of a male child at sunset. Wet cloths were placed upon the abdomen and the genital parts to prevent soreness and pain, and the body was partially cleansed soon after the birth. At about nine o'clock in the evening, a thorough ablution over the whole surface was practiced in a wash-tub, by a faithful nurse and the husband. She slept well during the night. Early in the morning a similar bath was again performed, the water about 70 degrees F. These baths were given four times a day generally; early in the morning, about an hour before dinner, ditto supper, and quite late at night on going to rest. The wet cloths about the abdomen, etc., were used a part of the time. Mrs. R. sat up a considerable portion of each day, lying down occasionally to rest herself. Every bath, she said, gave her new vigor. Thus alternating with bathing, reclining, and sitting up, there was no chance for her to become weaker than she was at the time of birth, but she in fact grew stronger every day. The third or fourth day she rode out, and could have done so much sooner, but she did not wish to *alarm* the neighbors. I allowed no persons to come to fatigue and excite her by talking, as persons are apt to do on such occasions, especially when a new mode of treatment is adopted. I told the patient that when she was wel. enough to go about like others, and she desired to see her neighbors, they might come, and not before; and some thought it very strange that she should be walking in the garden and riding out, while yet they could not be allowed to call upon her.

The above are the only two cases of childbirth we had at Oyster Bay during the past summer.

CASE III.

The following case of a clergyman's wife in this city, was given by herself for the Water-Cure Journal, some months since:

"MR. EDITOR—I feel that I am under obligations to you, and a duty I owe the public, if you think best, to make known the happy effects I received from following your directions, previous to, during, and after my accouchement last August. On Wednesday, the 23d August, 1848, at half-past 12, noon, I presented my husband with a fine boy, with comparatively little suffering. I had one of the best physicians with me, and although allopathic in practice, he did not interfere with your advice. After the birth of the child, I had wet towels applied around my hips, etc.; at two P. M. I partook of peaches and milk, with Graham bread; remained comfortable till six o'clock P. M., when, with the assistance of my husband, being very weak, I got into a tub of water, and after being well bathed and rubbed, I found, on leaving my bath and investing myself with a wet girdle, that I could have walked across the room without assistance; but I merely walked to the bed, and soon sank into a sweet sleep, in which I remained until morning. The babe also slept all nigh. without waking. The

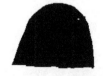

next morning, Thursday, the 24th, at six, I got up, took a bath, walked across the room to the rocking-chair, took my babe, and made him comfortable, for I thought I would not disturb him by dressing him. At twelve, twenty-four hours from the birth, I took another bath, and sat up till six, when I repeated the bath, and went to bed, and as I had eaten a very hearty dinner, I thought it best to deprive myself of supper. Friday morning, the 25th, I again took my bath early, had the windows of my rooms thrown open, and walked several times through them, and felt as well as ever, excepting a soreness across me, and weakness; had my bath at twelve; after dinner had some severe after-pains, but by constantly wearing the wet girdle, they were much alleviated, and soon ceased entirely.

"Saturday morning, the 26th, I again took the bath early, and exercised about the room; and after breakfast, which consisted of tomatoes, boiled corn, and potatoes, I washed and dressed my infant without feeling the least fatigue. I sat up most of this day—ate beans and corn for dinner. Sunday, 27th, I was so well that all the family went to church, leaving me with the babe and my little boy, five years old.

"When my child was a week old, I could go about the house, walk in the yard, and had read several volumes. I continued to take my baths and wear the wet girdle for six weeks, when I left them off on account of a journey I made to visit my parents in a distant city. I have delayed writing you to this time to see if we (the babe and myself) should continue in our favored state, and I have the pleasure of informing you that my health still remains good, and our babe is as well and fine as the fondest mother could wish.

" Now, when we take into consideration that I had no
nurse, nor had I to call on my girl for assistance during
the whole of my confinement, I think we may well ask
ourselves the question, How has it happened that what
has been heretofore considered a serious, and even dangerous event in the mother's life, should have all its ter-
rors, pains, and sickness, often attended with fatal fevers,
taken away, and reduced to a comparatively trifling
affair ?   I answer, and my experience warrants me in
answering (for I have had children before), *By the use
of cold water*, applied in a judicious manner ; a remedy
equally accessible to the poor as to the rich—simple,
vivifying, and effectual ; and I hope and trust you will
succeed in your very useful undertaking, and have the
happiness of conferring the same benefit on thousands
of trembling, anxious mothers, that you have on your
greatly obliged friend,   SARAH B."

CASE IV.

The case we here give, was written out by a medical
friend and college mate, who is now a missionary and
physician in a far distant country, and who is adopting
the water practice in connection with other modes.   His
education, both in general literature and medicine, is
much above that of the average of medical men.   His
opinions, therefore, should have the more weight on that
account.

" *March* 19*th*, 1846.—Desirous of availing myself of
an opportunity which the kindness of my friend, Dr.
Shew, afforded me—of witnessing the hydropathic treatment of cases of labor—I accompanied him to No. —
Second street, where he had been summoned a few

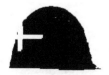

minutes before to attend a Mrs S., who was then in need of his services.

" Found the patient—an intelligent woman of the nervous temperament—with her constitution much broken down, though she was but 31 years of age, by the results of seven previous labors—the last a miscarriage. After some of her former confinements, she had been weeks and months in recovering; in one case, when she was treated fc. puerperal fever, her husband paid, in a single year, not less than $150 (no trifling sum out of the earnings of a working man with a large family) to the apothecary alone, for leeches and medicine. The patient had always been in the habit of using strong coffee and tea; drank the *mineral* water of the city wells; for some months past had relished nothing but the little delicacies sent in by her friends; and throughout the winter had been able to do little or no work at home.

" In consequence of excessive fatigue a few days before in ' house-hunting,' as she called it, she had been seized on Tuesday, the 17th, at 10 a. m., at the close of the fifth month of her gestation, with the pains of labor,—her former miscarriage having of course induced a predisposition to another. These pains increased in frequency and severity till they caused the greatest suffering, and prevented all sleep on Wednesday night and Thursday, up to the hour (3 p. m.) when she sent for Dr. S.

Here then was a patient whose previous history, impaired constitution, loss of sleep, and exhaustion from intense and almost incessant suffering, protracted now for more than two days, seemed to promise any thing but a *speedy* recovery, even should delivery be safely effected. It should be added, that *up to this time*, she

was an *utter stranger* even to the hydropathic regi
men.

"Her bowels having been moved the day before, all
that was deemed necessary was to render the condition
of the patient more comfortable by resorting to sedative
frictions along the spine with a towel wrung out of cold
water, and to the tepid hip bath, with sponging and rubbing the whole surface of the body. After this, less
complaint was made, till soon after 6 P. M. there was a
sudden aggravation of the bearing-down pains, resulting
in the delivery of a well-formed but still-born male child
of apparently five months.

"In about fifteen minutes the after-birth was detached
and taken away. Not over the usual amount of hæmorrhage occurred. A bandage was applied to the abdomen, as the patient expressed a wish for it; and after
resting awhile, a little panada was given to her as nourishment.

"Mrs. S. continued very comfortable through the evening; no excess of the lochial discharge; complained
only of exhaustion and slight dysuria. As some heat
of surface, pulse 90 to 100, tepid sponging resorted to,
which proved very grateful to the patient.

"*1st Day after Confinement (Friday)*, 7 *A. M.*—Found
patient had obtained considerable sleep at intervals during the night; felt very comfortable, though occasionally had slight pains in the abdomen; tongue moist,
pulse 81; had passed a little water during the night,
but with difficulty; had a strong desire for a cup of
coffee, but persuaded to take a little panada in its place.
Had not much appetite. Was permitted to sit up for a
few minutes while her bed was made.

"11½ *A. M.*—Mrs. S. still very comfortable; found

her sitting up in her rocking-chair, the very picture of convalescence ; pulse 80. Spong'ng enjoined, if any feverishness should arise

"3 *P. M.*—Dr. S. sent for, as the patient had been seized a few minutes before, rather suddenly, with a sharp pain on the left side of the hypogastric region. Had been drinking a tumbler of cold lemonade. Had a natural movement of the bowels that morning, and passed a little water. The tepid sponging of surface had been neglected. Pain—fixed, severe, pretty constant—remitting only for a moment or so. No corresponding contractions of uterine tumor observed. Some pain also complained of in the hip—in which she had on a former occasion been troubled. Up to that time had had no chill. Warm fomentations were applied, but with little relief.

"4½ *P. M.*—A chillness felt, then shivering, prolonged, with increase of the fixed pain in hypogastrium ; pulse 112, weak ; patient restless ; anxious, desponding, knitting of the brows ; involuntary weeping. A bottle of hot water was applied to the feet, and soon after the chill ceased.

"A large warm enema was now administered; brought away considerable of fœcal matter ; and fomentations were applied to the abdomen. Next the patient was seated in the hip bath, at a temperature of 95 degrees, for fifteen minutes, when water was passed more freely than before, ånd a slight nausea experienced. The result of this was complete abatement, for a time, of the pain in the uterine region, the diminution of the frequency of the pulse to 90, and great comfort. The bandage to abdomen having been removed to allow of the bath, was not replaced. If need be, fomentations to be kept up.

10

"At 7 p. m., found patient in a profuse perspiration; pain in abdomen had lost its acuteness; *soreness* there was all now complained of; soreness in head, ' in bones, and all over.' Abdomen tympanitic, tender on pressure, breathing thoracic; pulse 110—112; the lochial discharge arrested. Patient is to be kept quiet; to take no nourishment; no fire to be in the room.

"At 9¼ p. m., the perspiration still continues; complains ' pain in hip, but chiefly in the left part of the hypogastrium, as before, shooting across abdomen; pain very severe, increased by coughing; breathing thoracic, 28 in a minute; pulse 98; is thirsty; tongue moist, with a slight milky coat. Fomentations used.

" 10½ *P. M.*—Pain increasing in abdomen and hip; tenderness increasing; can scarce bear slightest pressure on abdomen, knees drawn up, restless, discouraged; pulse 100, though not very full or strong. Skin still moist, slightly.

"In this critical state of things, when nearly every symptom of that fearful disease, puerperal fever, was invading the system, and when, according to the prescribed rules of practice, the most vigorous antiphlogistic measures would be called for, a plan of treatment was adopted by Dr. Shew, which, as it seemed to me far more calculated to *kill* than to *cure*, I could not but protest against at the time, but which, as the result proved, was eminently calculated to turn back the tide of disease so rapidly setting in. It certainly affords striking evidence of the resources of Hydropathy, and its promptness and efficiency in relieving pain and extinguishing inflammation.

" Mrs. S. was carefully lifted from her bed, and after being placed awhile in her chair, was transferred to a hip bath containing about one pail of water fresh from the Croton hydrant near by, of the temperature of 42 degrees F. A towel wrung out of cold water was applied to her forehead at the same time. Of course, she was well covered with blankets. She had been seated thus but a few minutes when she expressed herself as feeling *very comfortable indeed*. The *severe pain* in her abdomen and thigh *had left her as if by magic*, and so complete was the relief that she fell into a gentle doze, from which, awakened by nodding, she observed, ' There, I feel so easy now, I lost myself, I believe.'

" While in the bath, her pulse was lowered several beats in a minute ; the unimmersed parts of the body remained warm ; the hips were to her of a refreshing coolness. After remaining thus seated in the water about twenty-five minutes, a slight addition of more cold water, by gradual pouring, having been made during this time, she was lifted back to the bed. Her pain had now entirely vanished ; the natural lochial discharge was soon restored ; her pulse reduced to 94 ; and, warm and comfortable, she had a prospect of a good night's rest.

" *2d Day (Saturday)*, 7 *A. M.*—Found patient looking comfortable and happy. No pain now in abdomen, slight soreness only ; tympanitis gone ; tongue moist and hardly coated ; pulse 79 ; had had no sensation of chilliness after her bath, but slept from 12½ to 4 A. M., without waking, and another doze after that : window had been a little raised all night, and no fire in the room, though a cool night. Now was able to pass water without difficulty. Was directed to take for breakfast some of the coarse bran bread toasted, and softened with milk, and a little scraped apple, if she wished.

" *Second Day after Confinement (Saturday)*, 11 *A. M.*

—Mrs. S. appears to be very comfortable. With the aid of a friend, had been up and changed her clothing Pulse 84, complains of no pain of any consequence in the abdomen.

" 1¼ *P. M.*—Having been under necessity of getting up without assistance, had fatigued herself, and thus induced a return of very severe pain in the uterine region. Dr. S. was sent for, when resort was had again to the hip bath, filled with cold water from the hydrant, which had with such wonderful promptitude averted the danger of puerperal fever, with which she was threatened on the evening of the previous day. As on that occasion, in less than five minutes the pain and feverishness was completely quelled. She was allowed to remain in the bath half an hour, and requested to abstain from food till evening.

" 5 *P. M.*—Patient doing remarkably well, cheerful— free from pains in abdomen, save now and then a very slight one ; some soreness on pressure ; pulse 84, compressible.

" 10 *P. M.*—Had slept during evening—had taken a little nourishment. As some difficulty in passing water, and as occasional slight pains and soreness still continued in the abdomen, the cold hip bath, temperature 42 F., was again resorted to for about thirty minutes. During this time the pulse was lowered from 80 beats in a minute to 70 ; water was passed freely, and the pains put to flight.

" After it, the patient continuing warm and comfortable—was directed, should there be any return of pains during the night, to seat herself in the hip bath, which was left in the room.

" *3d day* (*Sunday*), 7½ *A. M.*—Patient had slept most

of the night—looks bright—feels 'very comfortable'—pulse 72, soft and natural ; had raised herself in bed without difficulty and washed. On account of some dysuria, the hip bath was used for about fifteen minutes, when water was passed more freely and copiously than at any previous time.   Left seated in the rocking-chair, sitting up occasionally ; she says it has rested and re freshed her from the first.

"Appetite good—thinks even the plainest food would be relished.   Breakfast to be as before—the toasted coarse bread soaked in milk, with a little scraped apple. Directed to take no nourishment at any time unless a decided appetite, nor then oftener than three times a day. Is to take an enema and another hip bath in the course of the morning.

"6, *P. M.*—Had continued to gain during the day— till, toward evening, it most unfortunately happened that an intoxicated man, mistaking the house, strayed into the room where she was lying, with no attendant but a young girl ; seating himself without any ceremony in the rocking-chair, with a lighted cigar in his mouth, he smoked away to his satisfaction, and then very deliber-ately composed himself for a nap.   This strange visitor and the fumes of the tobacco had given poor Mrs. S. a severe headache, the first with which she had been troubled—considerable nausea with paleness of face— cold feet, etc. A towel wet with cold water was ap-plied to the head, and a hip bath ordered.

"*Half past 9, P. M.*—Was rapidly recovering from the effects of the afternoon's unexpected visit—sat up a while.

"*Fourth day, Monday.*—At 7½ A. M. found Mrs. S. sitting up in bed, sewing—pulse 75—had rested well—

10*

has a good appetite. Breakfast to be as before—may safely take a hip bath any time when suffers from pain and is not made chilly by sitting in it.

"Was able this morning to rise and walk about the room unsupported. Required no assistance in getting to the bath, bowels moved naturally—sat up several hours to-day, appears bright, pleasant, and cheerful.

"*Fifth day, Tuesday.*—Mrs. S. 'feels to-day as much better than she did yesterday, as she did yesterday better than the day before.' Sat up, and was about the room nearly all day—continues the practice of daily sponging of whole surface and the use of the hip bath At night retention having ensued from over-distention of the bladder, in consequence of an untimely protracted visit from some of patient's friends, Dr. S. was sent for. and deemed it advisable to resort to the catheter, which she had frequently been compelled to use on former occasions, sometimes for months together.

"*Sixth day, Wednesday.*—Mrs. S. appeared to be better in the morning—able to rise without assistance, to walk about, and even to sweep the room; catheter again required.

"*Seventh day, Thursday.*—During the night, of her own accord, took three or four cool hip baths, and found them refreshing and of service in promoting easy evacuation of the bladder. At one time dropped asleep, and remained so an hour or more, sitting in the water. Pulse in the morning 62. Dressed the children, and arranged the room herself to-day—and though a week had hardly elapsed since her confinement, felt *strong enough in the morning to go down stairs* and to do a half day's work in sewing, etc., from which she appeared to experience no injury. A few days afte: she ventured to ride down to the lower part of the city, and having since continued to improve, save an occasional return of an old difficulty, retention—is most gratefully sensible of her indebtedness, under heaven, to her physician and Hydropathy for a far more speedy and pleasant convalescence than she ever experienced after any of her former confinements."

If the limits of this work permitted, I might give scores of cases which have occurred either in my own practice or come under my immediate observation during the past six years, in which the results were, on an average, as favorable as in those we have given. But this is not necessary. I have given enough to serve as a general guide to the treatment. Nor would I, for any consideration, be the means of misleading people in this important matter of childbirth. I am fully convinced that those persons who will follow out the rules I have here laid down, for fortifying and invigorating the general health, will arrive at results similar to those I have described. And I am stimulated in my labors in this department, by the firm belief that many a suffering woman will feel grateful for the information which I have imparted.

I will here remark, that bathing during the time of labor may prove as useful as when the patient is much exhausted from pain and the expulsive efforts. Perhaps it would be well sometimes to use the hip bath. By this means the contractions of the womb would be greater, and I think with less pain. I have not as yet been in the habit of directing this application in more than a few instances. It is a safe means, and those can resort to it who choose. I would not, however, recommend them to be taken for more than ten or fifteen minutes at a time. Some have taken them for hours at a time, and during the most of the labor. But such a practice, although it may not result in positive harm at the time ought not to be employed.

Cold water injections in the bowels are often useful in causing the pains to become more efficient during labor. By this means, also, the lower bowel is thoroughly emptied, and thus more room is left for the passage of the child. The freeing of the bowels at or just before labor should always be attended to.

CHAPTER VIII.

CONCLUSION.

Management after Childbirth.—Popular objections answered.—The evils of Confinement in Bed.—The injurious Effects of the common Bandage or Binder.—The use of cold Water and the wet Girdle in all respects better Means.—After-Pains.—How to be prevented.—Swelling of the Breasts.—Cold Water a sovereign Remedy.—Sore Nipples.—Injections after Labor.—Management of the Child.—When to separate the Umbilical Cord.—The best mode of washing the Infant.—The common Bandage not to be Applied.—Very important Advice as regards weaning and feeding Infants.

MANAGEMENT AFTER CHILDBIRTH.

THE truly remarkable effects of water-treatment in enabling our patients to recover so soon from the effects of childbirth, meets with great opposition on the part of some of the medical fraternity. Falling of the womb, it is said, must often be the inevitable result of persons getting about so soon. It should be remembered, that this calamity comes in consequence of *general debility*; and if we cause our patients to go about too much and too soon after childbirth, so as to cause a sufficient degree of general debility, then this result would necessarily follow such a course. But the truth is, the danger lies on the other side. Does not every mother who has been attended in the way of the old modes, know that some days after delivery, they become more debilitated than at the time of the birth? The reason by which to account for this is the bad treatment practiced. Lying constantly in bed, even for a single day only, will make a strong person weak, nervous, and restless. How much more, then, if the practice is continued for days! In a properly managed water-treatment, the patient grows day by day more strong, and for this reason falling of the womb is not so liable to occur as in the old modes. There is far greater danger in the latter than the former.

THE BINDER OR BANDAGE

The universal use of the obstetrical bandage or binder after delivery, is practiced on the assumption that nature is incompetent to do her own work. It is true that art must sometimes be brought to assist her in her operations, but such is not the rule. As the bandage is generally applied, it is almost certain of slipping upward, thus tending to cause one of the very evils—falling of the womb—which it is intended to prevent. Besides, it heats the body too much, thereby causing general debility, a greater tendency to after pains, constipation, and puerperal fever. If it is ever used, it should be only in those cases where the debility is very great, and then only a portion of the time. The constringing and invigorating effect of cold water upon the muscles of the abdomen renders those patients who use it, not only as good, but of a better form than those who use the common bandage. I speak from positive knowledge in this matter, not from mere theory alone.

The common wet girdle, which is explained elsewhere in this work, may be worn either a part or the whole of the time after confinement; and the same general rules for its use apply here as elsewhere.

AFTER-PAINS.

After-pains are caused by clots of blood accumulating within the cavity of the womb. Persons of high nervous susceptibility sometimes suffer exceedingly with these pains; more even than at the time of labor. In such cases, bathing should be persevered in, hourly, if need be, until the pains are literally worried out. The cold rubbing wet-sheet is here an excellent remedy. Cold injections to the bowels are also good, and may be as often repeated as is desired. The bath by means of sitting in a wash-tub, may also be employed.

SWELLING OF THE BREASTS.

There is necessarily more or less excitement of the system as the milk begins to secrete. The breasts and nipples should be kept perfectly clean, and should be washed at least two or three times daily in cold water. Nothing in the world is so good to prevent that troublesome affection, soreness of the nipples, as washing them often, both before and after labor, in cold water. If the breasts inflame, the heat must be kept down by pouring cold water freely upon them, and the use of the wet cloths. No poultices are so good as these. In the water-treatment, properly managed, we have never to encounter that most painful and troublesome affection, breaking or abscess of the breasts.

Mothers cannot be too careful in keeping the breasts at all times well drawn.

INJECTIONS AFTER LABOR.

Some writers have advocated that the bowels should be kept in a quiescent state, if they be so inclined, as is often the case, for some days after labor. But this is not a good rule. To leave the bowels inactive, tends to cause feverishness—the circumstance most to be feared after the confinement. See that the bowels act at least once every day. The morning, before eating, is on the whole the most suitable time. But if after-pains are troublesome, the cold injection may be repeated often during the day. Injections on going to rest, often have a good effect as regards sleep.

MANAGEMENT OF THE CHILD.

The umbilical cord should never be separated from the child until the pulsations of its arteries have entirely ceased. This will usually require not more than ten or fifteen minutes, perhaps generally not so long.

Very soon after birth the child should be well washed in water of moderate temperature. About 80 degrees F. in summer, and 70 degrees in winter, will, I think, be as good a rule as could be given. If necessary, a little mild soap may be used. It is better, however, to get along without it. A little lard rubbed upon the sur face many prefer ; some get along without any thing but simple water.

No bandage should be put about the abdomen of the new-born child. The practice of girting up infants until they can scarcely breathe, is a barbarism that is destined soon to die away. Some thicknesses of fine wet linen may from time to time be placed over the navel as a poultice, after it begins to become sore. The navel heals much sooner with the water dressing than with such as are generally used. The form of the infant's abdomen, treated without the bandage, is, to say the least, as good as when treated with it. We repeat, the common practice of girting children after birth is a cruel one, that ought never to be tolerated.

I do not believe in using very cold water for the daily ablutions of infants. It does no good to make them blue by bathing. An infant that is nursed properly, and kept from over-heated rooms, and all great changes and extremes in temperature, needs only bathing enough for cleanliness. A morning and evening washing, with at other times proper cleansing of parts soiled by the natural discharges, will, as a rule, be all that is required. No feather beds or pillows should be allowed for infants, The heat engendered by these always renders them more feeble and liable to colds.

I will close by giving one piece of advice, which I trust will be of incalculable service to all who choose to follow it—namely, in regard to the feeding of children. It is very common with mothers to commence early feeding their infants solid food. I believe many a child is destroyed in this way. If in case it is necessary to feed an infant with other food than that best of all, the mother's milk, give it cow's milk, without any addition at all, except, if it be very rich, an eight or tenth part of pure water may be added to it. Not a particle of sugar or any thing else. It should be fed slowly with a small spoon, or some other contrivance, but never faster than it could get it at nurse. I believe, too, that children are weaned much too young as a general thing in this country. The teeth should be well formed before weaning. And after this, solid food must be commenced with the greatest caution, or bowel complaint will most certainly ensue. Remember adult persons may live well, and be cured of a great variety of diseases, by being restricted wholly to cow's milk, about two quarts per day. The milk should not be boiled; but as to whether it is better to warm it for a very young infant or not, I do not know. Infants do well with cold milk. If the application of heat to raise it to the temperature of the mother's milk causes no chemical change, by which it is injured, that would perhaps be the better mode.*

* Since writing the above paragraphs, I notice in a work entitled " Physical Education and the preservation of Health," by Dr. Warren, the elder and distinguished surgeon of Boston, the following advice : " The food of young infants should be administered to them at stated periods, and not whenever they cry. Children very frequently cry from having taken too much food. A good rule for general use is, to give nourishment to the child once in about three hours. From the time of weaning until the first dentition is over, their best food is bread and milk ; coarse bread is better than fine in most cases."

This advice is, on the whole, very good ; but how are we to determine in which the coarse bread is best and in which the fine ? I regard that the same great law holds good in all cases. Whenever it is proper at all to give solid food, the coarse bread will be *in all cases* the best.

It is doubtful, also, whether bread of any kind is as good as well-boiled rice for the first solid food to be given the infant. At all events, rice *is* an excellent article. And the same may be said of white Indian meal, very thoroughly boiled. Thus prepared, Indian meal is a light article, and agrees well with young children ; poorly prepared, it is a very bad article.

I still believe, however, as stated in the text, that either the mother's milk, or that of a healthy cow, is preferable to all solid food until the first teeth are well formed. Teething of itself is hard enough for the child to endure, without adding to its dangers that of weaning, or the change to solid food.

INDEX.

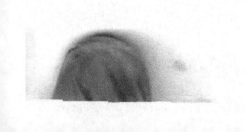

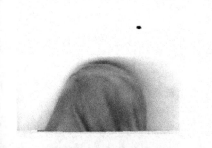

Check Out More Titles From HardPress Classics Series In this collection we are offering thousands of classic and hard to find books. This series spans a vast array of subjects — so you are bound to find something of interest to enjoy reading and learning about.

Subjects:
Architecture
Art
Biography & Autobiography
Body, Mind &Spirit
Children & Young Adult
Dramas
Education
Fiction
History
Language Arts & Disciplines
Law
Literary Collections
Music
Poetry
Psychology
Science
…and many more.

Visit us at www.hardpress.net

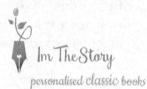
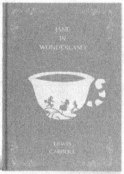